ORGANON
OF
MEDICINE

ORGANON
OF
MEDICINE

SAMUEL HAHNEMANN

THE FIRST INTEGRAL ENGLISH TRANSLATION
OF THE DEFINITIVE SIXTH EDITION OF THE ORIGINAL
WORK ON HOMOEOPATHIC MEDICINE

JOST KÜNZLI, M.D., ALAIN NAUDÉ, AND PETER PENDLETON

Cooper Publishing
Blaine, Washington

Organon of Medicine

Translation copyright © 1982 by Alain Naudé

ISBN 0-9636312-0-9 (previously ISBN 0-87477-223-0)

Cooper Publishing,
250 H St., PO Box 2187,
Blaine, Washington 98231
United States of America

PRINTED IN CANADA

Reprinted in 1996

Library of Congress cataloged a previous edition as follows:

Hahnemann, Samuel, 1755-1843.
    The organon of medicine.

    Translation of Organon der rationellen Heilkunde.
    Includes index.
    1. Homoeopathy. I. Title.
RX68.O513 1982   615.5'32   82-3244
ISBN 0-87477-222-2 (Cloth)   AACR2
ISBN 0-87477-223-0 (Paper)

Translators' Introduction

Samuel Hahnemann's *Organon of Medicine* clearly and completely states, for the first time in history, the true nature of health and disease, the natural principles of cure, and the system of medical therapy based on these principles which we know as homoeopathy. It has remained until today the one essential cornerstone of homoeopathy, the ultimate authority on its doctrine and practice. Everything ever written on homoeopathy proceeds from it.

It was first published in 1810, in Köthen, Germany. Hahnemann published five editions of the work during his lifetime and completed the manuscript of the sixth and final edition in 1842, the year before he died at the age of eighty-eight. This last edition was not published until 1921.

The standard English version of the *Organon* has hitherto been a nineteenth-century translation of the fifth edition, to which a translation of the important changes introduced by Hahnemann in the sixth edition were later added in an effort to bring it up to date. Unfortunately, this translation is very tedious and difficult to read because it approximates in stilted Victorian English the dense and cumbersome style of Hahnemann's German. Hahnemann's language is difficult even for a modern German ear, and its literal equivalent in English is a formidable obstacle to understanding. Furthermore, there are serious errors in the translation and in the additions made to it.

The present translators have made a completely new translation from the original text of the sixth edition. Hahnemann's manuscript is in the possession of the School of Medicine of the University of California in San Francisco, and we have been fortunate in obtaining a photocopy of it. We have scrupulously adhered to every word of Hahnemann's text but have rendered it into standard modern English, sometimes dividing his very long sentences into several shorter ones for the sake of clarity and readability.

There has been a most remarkable reawakening of interest in homoeopathy during the last ten years, and many important textbooks have been republished in different English-speaking countries. It seemed therefore all the more urgent to bring out a clear English translation of the book from which all others in the literature developed and on which they comment.

This translation is the fruit of many months of arduous labor; it has been rigorously and systematically checked against the original text by us and by other scholars. It was commissioned by The Hahnemann Foundation of California with the intention of providing a reliable modern English source for homoeopathic physicians and the public.

The *Organon* may in time be widely recognized as one of the most important books in the entire history of medicine, because it introduces in the long story of man's struggle against disease a successful system of medicinal therapy that contrasts radically with everything previously taught and practiced.

Homoeopathy is recognized and practiced throughout the world, but it is still something of a challenge to the orthodox medical establishment, which can neither assimilate it nor refute it.

Amid the public doubts and criticisms that today cloud the image of technological medicine, homoeopathy offers a clear, simple, and inexpensive way to cure disease. It may indeed turn out to be the new medicine of the world.

Jost Künzli, M.D.
Alain Naudé
Peter Pendleton

Acknowledgments

We would like to express our deep gratitude to the following, without whom our task could not have been completed: Richard Trapp, chairman of the Department of Classics, San Francisco State University, for translating the Latin passages in the text; Elinor Roos, for painstakingly preparing an excellent index to this work; Nicoletta Mustart, for her many hours of typing and conscientious proofreading; Mary Lutyens, for reading the final manuscript; and all the other faithful friends of homoeopathy in different parts of the world who have helped with their encouragement and support.

We dedicate this translation of the
Organon *to its author, Samuel*
Hahnemann, with love and respect, and
hope that he would have found it worthy.

Organon of Medicine

Samuel Hahnemann

1

The physician's highest calling, his *only* calling, is to make sick people healthy—to heal, as it is termed.[a]

a. It is not to weave so-called systems from fancy ideas and hypotheses about the inner nature of the vital processes and the origin of diseases in the invisible interior of the organism (on which so many fame-seeking physicians have wasted their powers and time). Nor does it consist of trying endlessly to explain disease phenomena and their proximate cause, which will always elude him.

Nor does it consist of holding forth in unintelligible words or abstract and pompous expressions in an effort to appear learned so as to astonish the ignorant, while the world in sickness cries in vain for help.

Surely by now we have had enough of these pretentious fantasies called *theoretical medicine,* for which university chairs have even been established, and it is time for those calling themselves physicians to stop deceiving poor human beings by their talk and to *start acting instead*—that is, really helping and healing.

2

The highest ideal of therapy is to restore health rapidly, gently, permanently; to remove and destroy the whole disease in the shortest, surest, least harmful way, according to clearly comprehensible principles.

3

If the physician clearly perceives what has to be cured in disease, i.e., in each individual case of disease (*knowledge of the disease*),

if he clearly perceives what it is in medicines which heals, i.e., in each individual medicine (*knowledge of medicinal powers*),

if he applies in accordance with well-defined principles what is curative in medicines to what he has clearly recognized to be pathological in the patient, so that cure follows, i.e., if he knows in each particular case how to apply the remedy most appropriate by its character (*selection of the remedy*), prepare it exactly as required and give it in the right amount (*the correct dose*), and repeat the dose exactly when required,

and, lastly, if in each case he knows the obstacles to cure and how to remove them, so that recovery is permanent,

then he knows how to treat thoroughly and efficaciously, and is a true physician.

4

The physician is likewise a preserver of health if he knows the things that disturb it, that cause and sustain illness, and if he knows how to remove them from healthy people.

5

In addition, it will help the physician to bring about a cure if he can determine the most probable *exciting cause* in an acute disease and the most significant phases in the evolution of a chronic, long-lasting disease, enabling him to discover its *underlying cause,* usually a chronic miasm.

In this he should consider: the evident physical constitution of the patient (especially in chronic affections), his affective and intellectual character, his activities, his way of life, his habits, his social position, his family relationships, his age, his sexual life, etc.

6

The unprejudiced observer realizes the futility of metaphysical speculations that cannot be verified by experiment, and no matter how clever he is, he sees in any given case of disease only the disturbances of body and soul which are perceptible to the senses: subjective symptoms, incidental symptoms, objective symptoms, i.e., deviations from the former healthy condition of the individual now sick which the patient personally feels, which people around him notice, which the physician sees in him.

The totality of these perceptible signs represents the entire extent of the sickness; together they constitute its true and only conceivable form.[a]

a. This is why I do not know how at the sickbed one can imagine that one has to seek out and can find what is to be cured in disease only in the hidden and unknowable interior of the human organism; how one can fail to pay most careful attention to symptoms and be scrupulously guided by them to cure. I do not know how one can be so ridiculous and presumptuous as to try to recognize what has changed in the depths of the body without paying special attention to the symptoms or how one can try to reestablish its order with medicines of which one knows nothing, calling this method the only radical and rational therapy.

As far as the physician is concerned, is not that which reveals itself to the senses in symptoms the very disease itself? He can never see the immaterial element, the vital force causing the disease. He need never see it; to cure he needs only to see and understand its morbific effects.

What kind of *prima causa morbi* is the old school looking for in the hidden depths of the body if it rejects and haughtily disdains the comprehensible and clearly perceptible manifestations of disease, i.e., the symptoms speaking in understandable language? What else do they want to cure in disease but these symptoms?

7

Since one may know a disease only by its symptoms, when there is no obvious exciting or sustaining cause (*causa occasionalis*) to be removed,[a] it is evident that only the symptoms, together with any possible miasm and additional circumstances, must guide the choice of the appropriate, curative medicine (par. 5).

So it is the totality of symptoms, *the outer image expressing the inner essence of the disease, i.e., of the disturbed vital force,* that must be the main, even the only, means by which the disease allows us to find the necessary remedy, the only one that can decide the appropriate choice.

Briefly, in every individual case of disease the totality of the symptoms[b] must be the physician's principal concern, the only object of his attention, the only thing to be *removed* by his intervention in order to cure, i.e., to transform the disease into health.

a. It is obvious that every reasonable physician will first of all remove the *causa occasionalis;* after that the indisposition usually disappears on its own. For instance, he removes from the sickroom the strong-smelling flowers that have brought on faintness and hysterical manifestations; he removes from the cornea the foreign body that is producing ophthalmia; he loosens and readjusts the tight bandage that threatens to cause gangrene in a wounded limb; he uncovers and ties the severed artery that is causing shock; he tries by emetics to void the Belladonna berries, etc., that have been swallowed; he removes the foreign objects introduced into the natural openings of the body (nose, throat, ears, urethra, rectum, vagina); he crushes the stones in the bladder; he opens the imperforate anus of the new-born infant, etc.

b. Usually not knowing what else to do, the old school has always tried to combat and wherever possible suppress through medicines *only one* of the many symptoms that diseases present—a *shortsighted method* called symptomatic therapy.

This has justly earned general contempt, not only because it does not do any real good but because it does much harm.

A single symptom is no more the whole disease than a single foot a whole man. This method is all the more objectionable because it treats a particular symptom with an opposite remedy (in a merely enantiopathic and palliative way) with the result that it returns much worse than before after a short alleviation.

8

After the elimination of all the symptoms and perceptible signs of disease, one cannot imagine or demonstrate by any experiment in the world that anything but health remains, that anything but health could remain; nor can one doubt that all the pathological changes inside the organism have been neutralized.[a]

a. When someone has been cured by a real physician, so that no sign or symptom of disease remains and all the indications of health have permanently returned, can one without affronting human intelligence possibly maintain that the disease continues to dwell somewhere in the economy?

Yet this is what a past authority of the old school, Hufeland, maintained when he said (*Homöopathie*, p. 27, l. 19): "Homoeopathy can remove symptoms, but the disease remains." He said this partly out of spite because of the progress of homoeopathy for the good of mankind and partly because of his still totally materialistic conception of disease. He could not conceive of it as a state of being of the organism dynamically untuned by a disturbed vital force, as an alteration in the state of health, but considered it as a *material thing,* which could, after a cure, remain hidden in some secret corner of the organism to reveal its material presence at a later date, breaking out at will right in the midst of flourishing health!

Such is as yet the blindness of the old pathology! After all that, no wonder it has no other therapy to offer than "sweeping clean" the poor patient!

9

In the state of health the spirit-like vital force (*dynamis*) animating the material human organism reigns in supreme sovereignty.

It maintains the sensations and activities of all the parts of the living organism in a harmony that obliges wonderment. The reasoning spirit who inhabits the organism can thus freely use this healthy living instrument to reach the lofty goal of human existence.

10

Without the vital force the material organism is unable to feel, or act, or maintain itself.[a] Only because of the immaterial being (vital principle, vital force) that animates it in health and in disease can it feel and maintain its vital functions.

a. Without the vital force the body dies; and then, delivered exclusively to the forces of the outer material world, it decomposes, reverting to its chemical constituents.

11

When man falls ill it is at first only this self-sustaining spirit-like vital force (vital principle) everywhere present in the organism which is untuned by the dynamic[a] influence of the hostile disease agent.

It is only this vital force thus untuned which brings about in the organism the disagreeable sensations and abnormal functions that we call *disease*. Being invisible, and recognizable solely by its effects on the organism, it can express itself and reveal its untunement only by pathological manifestations in feeling and function (the only aspects of the organism accessible to the senses of the observer and the physician), i.e., *disease symptoms*.

a. What is dynamic influence, dynamic force? We see that the earth causes the moon to revolve around it in twenty-eight days and a number of hours by some invisible mysterious force and that the moon in its turn produces in the ocean at regular intervals alternating tides of ebb and flow (with some variations at the full and the new moon). We see this and are amazed, because our senses do not realize how it happens. Obviously this is not produced by material means or by the mechanical contrivances of men. And we see about us a great many other events caused by the action of one substance upon another without being able to detect any visible sequence of cause and effect. Only a cultivated man accustomed to comparison and abstraction can intuitively form an idea of this phenomenon: upon reflection he sees it to be beyond material and mechanical influences. He terms it the *dynamic, virtual* action of forces, that which takes place by the absolute, specific, pure power that one force exerts upon another.

In the same way, the dynamic force with which pathogenetic influences act on healthy individuals and the *dynamic* force with which medicines act upon the vital principle to restore health are nothing but a contagion devoid of any material or mechanical aspect. A magnet powerfully attracts a piece of iron or steel near it in a similar way: one sees that the piece of iron is attracted by a pole of the magnet but does *not* see *how* this takes place. The invisible force of the magnet does not need any mechanical (material) means, such as a hook or lever; it attracts the iron or a steel needle by its own pure, nonmaterial, invisible, spirit-like force. We have here a *dynamic* phenomenon. Moreover, it invisibly (dynamically) transmits magnetic force to the steel needle, which in turn becomes magnetic even without being touched by the magnet, even at some distance, and is then able to transmit the same magnetic quality to other steel needles (dynamically).

In a similar way a child who has smallpox or measles will transmit them to a healthy child by approaching him, even without touching him. This contamination takes place invisibly (dynamically) at a distance, with no more transmission of any material particle from one to the other than from the magnet to the steel needle. A specific, spirit-like influence communicates smallpox or measles to the child nearby, just as the magnet communicates magnetic force to the needle.

The action of medicines upon living people must be judged in a similar way. Natural substances that have been found to be medicinal are so only by virtue of their power (specific to each one of them) to modify the human organism through a dynamic, spirit-like effect (transmitted through sensitive living tissue) upon the spirit-like vital principle that governs life.

Those natural substances that in a narrower sense we call medicines are so only because they have the power to bring about changes in animal life. These medicinal substances capable of acting on the organism exert their nonmaterial (dynamic) influence only on the spirit-like vital force. In the same way the magnetic pole communicates to the steel needle, as if by contagion, *only* magnetic force and not other qualities, such as increased hardness or malleability, etc.

Thus any particular medicine will change the condition of a person's health (by a sort of contagion) in its own specific way and not in the way some other medicine would act, just as certainly as the proximity of a child with smallpox will communicate to a healthy child smallpox and never measles.

The influence of medicines upon our organism is exerted *dynamically,* as if by contagion, without the transmission of the slightest particle of the material medicinal substance.

When indicated, the smallest dose of a properly dynamized medicine—in which calculation shows that there is only an infinitesimal amount of material substance left, so little that it cannot be imagined or conceived by the best mathematicians—exerts *far* more healing power than strong material doses of the same medicine. This very subtle dose, which contains almost nothing but the spirit-like medicinal force released and freed, can bring about, solely by its *dynamic* power, results impossible to obtain with crude medicinal substances, even in massive doses.

The specific invisible medicinal force of these highly potentized remedies does not depend on their material atoms or on their physical surfaces—ideas that are the product of useless and still materialistic theorizing about the higher power of potentized remedies. On the contrary, it is the invisible energy of the crude substance released and freed to the highest possible extent which is to be found in the minute impregnated globule or its solution. Upon contact with living tissue, this medicinal force acts dynamically on the whole organism in a specific way, without communicating to it the smallest material particle, however subtle; and it does so more and more powerfully as it becomes freer and less material through progressive dynamization (par. 270).

In our time, which boasts such enlightened and deepthinking souls, does it have to be so impossible to conceive of a nonmaterial dynamic force when we see around us every day so many phenomena that cannot be explained in any other way? Is it through taking substantial doses of an emetic to bring about antiperistaltic movements in the stomach that we feel nausea at the sight of something sickening? Is it not exclusively the dynamic action of seeing something revolting upon our imagination? Do we need a lever or a visible material contraption to lift an arm? Is it not exclusively the nonmaterial dynamic force of the will which lifts it?

12

It is only the pathologically untuned vital force that causes diseases.[a]

The pathological manifestations accessible to our senses express all the internal changes, i.e., the whole pathological disturbance of the *dynamis:* they reveal the whole disease.

Conversely, the cessation through treatment of all the symptoms, i.e., the disappearance of all perceptible deviations from health, necessarily implies that the vital principle has recovered its integrity and therefore that the whole organism has returned to health.

a. How does the vital force bring the organism to produce symptoms, i.e., *how* does it make disease? Such questions are of no value to the physician. The answers will always be hidden from him. The Master and Lord of life has revealed to his senses only what is necessary and completely sufficient to cure diseases.

13

It follows that disease (excluding surgical cases) is not, as the allopaths believe:

an entity, however subtle, hidden in the interior of the organism separate from its living totality;

or an entity separate from the vital force, from the dynamic power that gives life to the organism.

Such a phantom[a] can be conceived only by materialistic minds. It is this phantom that has for millennia pushed official medicine along the deadly road it has traveled, making it an art of darkness incapable of healing.

a. Materia peccans!

14

There is no curable disease or morbific alteration hidden in the interior of the body which does not announce itself to the conscientiously observant physician through objective and subjective symptoms. This is what the omniscient Preserver of.human life has provided in his infinite goodness.

15

In the invisible interior of the body, the suffering of the pathologically untuned spirit-like *dynamis* (vital force) animating the organism and the totality of perceptible symptoms that result and that represent the disease are one and the same.

The organism is the material instrument of life; but it is no more conceivable without the life-giving, regulating, instinctively feeling *dynamis* than this *dynamis* is conceivable without the organism. The two are one, even if thought separates them to facilitate comprehension.

16

Outer malefic agents that harm the healthy organism and disturb the harmonious rhythm of life can reach and affect the spirit-like *dynamis* only in a way that also is dynamic and spirit-like.

The physician can remove these pathological untunements (diseases) only by acting on our spirit-like vital force with medicines having equally spirit-like, dynamic[a] effects that are perceived by the nervous sensitivity everywhere present in the organism.

So it is only by dynamic action upon the vital principle that remedies can restore health and the harmony of life after the perceptible changes in health (the totality of symptoms) have revealed the disease to the carefully observing and inquiring physician fully enough to be cured.

[a]. See footnote to paragraph 11.

17

Cure, which is the elimination of all the perceptible signs and symptoms of disease, means also the removal of the inner modifications of the vital force which underlie them: in this way the whole disease has been destroyed.[a]

Consequently the physician has only to eliminate the totality of the symptoms in order to remove simultaneously the inner alteration, the pathological untunement of the vital principle, thereby entirely removing and annihilating the *disease itself.*[b]

Now, when disease is destroyed, health is restored, and this is the highest goal, the only goal of the physician who knows the significance of his calling, which is to help his fellow man, not to indulge in pretentious prattle.

[a]. It is possible to create a very grave disease by acting on the vital principle through the power of imagination and to cure it in the same way.

A prophetic dream, a superstitious fancy, or the solemn prediction of death on a certain day or at a certain hour have often produced all the worsening symptoms of disease, even to the point of leading one to expect early death—indeed, even to death itself at the predicted hour; this would not be possible without the simultaneous production of an inner change equal to the visible outer one.

By a similar influence, such as an artful pretense or a countersuggestion, it is often possible to banish all the signs announcing early death and to restore health promptly. This would not be possible if this exclusively psychological remedy did not remove the inner and outer disturbances leading to the expectation of death.

b. God, the Preserver of mankind, reveals his wisdom and goodness in the cure of sickness afflicting humanity by clearly showing the physician what he needs to remove in diseases in order to annihilate them and restore health. But what would we have to conclude about his wisdom and goodness if (as the old school maintains, affecting an oracular insight into the hidden nature of things) he had instead clouded in mysterious obscurity what has to be cured, locking it up inside and depriving the physician of the possibility of clearly recognizing the trouble and curing it?

18

It is an indubitable truth that there is absolutely nothing else but the totality of symptoms—including the concomitant circumstances of the case (par. 5)   by which a disease can express its need for help.

We can categorically declare that the *totality of symp-*

toms and circumstances observed in each individual
case is the one and only indication that can guide us to
the choice of the remedy.

19

Since *diseases* are only *deviations from the healthy
condition*, and since they express themselves through
symptoms, and since *cure* is equally only a *change from
the diseased condition* back to the state of *health*, one
easily sees that *medicines* can cure disease only if they
possess the power to alter the way a person feels and
functions. Indeed, it is *only* because of this power that
they are medicines.

20

It is impossible only through the efforts of the intel-
lect to recognize the spirit-like force itself, which, hidden in the intimate essence of the medicines, gives them
the power to change the way people feel and thereby to
cure diseases.

It is only through its effects on the human economy
that we may experience and clearly perceive it.

21

Beyond question, the curative essence of medicines
cannot be recognized in itself. Pure experiments conducted by even the most perceptive observer can reveal
nothing to explain why medicinal substances cure except
that they bring about evident changes in the human economy, specifically that they provoke a number of definite
symptoms in and upon the *healthy*. It follows that when
remedies cure they do so only through their ability to
alter human health by causing characteristic symptoms.

Therefore we should concern ourselves exclusively with the disease symptoms that medicines bring about in the healthy, the only means by which they reveal their inherent curative virtues, to discover each one's disease-producing power and thereby its curative power.

22

To change diseases into health the only thing that must be removed is the totality of the subjective and objective symptoms.

The curative power of medicines consists exclusively in their propensity to produce disease symptoms in the healthy and remove them from the sick.

It follows on the one hand that substances become remedies and are able to destroy disease only by arousing certain manifestations and symptoms, i.e., particular artificial disease conditions, which are capable of eliminating and destroying the symptoms that already exist, i.e., the natural disease being treated; and, conversely, that for the totality of symptoms to be cured, one must seek that medicine which has demonstrated the greatest propensity to produce either *similar* or *opposite* symptoms.

Now, whether to treat disturbances with *similar* or with *opposite* medicinal symptoms to remove existing disease symptoms and restore health as gently, surely, and permanently as possible is something that only experiment will reveal.[a]

a. In addition to these two possible modes of treatment there is a third, the *allopathic method,* which prescribes medicines having symptoms with no direct pathic relationship to the disease condition, symptoms neither similar nor opposite but completely heterogeneous.

As I have stated elsewhere, this method plays with the life of the patient irresponsibly and murderously, with its massive doses of dangerously violent drugs of unknown action chosen upon mere conjecture, its painful procedures that are supposed to divert sickness to other parts, its exhaustion of the patient by emptying him from above and from below, by making him sweat or salivate, but worst of all, in accordance with the present fashion, by blindly and relentlessly wasting his irreplaceable blood. . . . All this is done on the pretext that the physician has to imitate and assist the efforts that diseased nature makes to restore itself, and without the understanding that it is senseless to try to imitate and assist the very imperfect and most often inappropriate efforts of the purely instinctive and unreasoning vital force. The vital force was given to us to sustain our life in harmony as long as we are healthy, not to heal itself when diseased, for if it possessed an ability so worthy of imitation, it would never allow the organism to fall ill.

When afflicted by disease agents, our vital force can express its untunement only through disturbances in the normal functions of the organism and through pain, whereby it calls for the help of a wise physician. If such help is not forthcoming, it tries to save itself at all costs by increasing the suffering and especially by violent evacuations, often at the cost of tremendous sacrifice, sometimes at the cost of life itself.

The pathologically untuned vital force has so little abilty to cure that it certainly does not deserve to be imitated, since all the symptoms and changes it produces in the organism are precisely the disease itself! Would any reasonable physician who is unwilling to sacrifice his patient try to imitate it in order to cure?

23

All carefully conducted experimentation and research prove to us that persistent disease symptoms, far from being wiped out and destroyed by opposite medicinal symptoms (in the *antipathic, enantiopathic,* or *palliative method*), return instead with renewed intensity and evident aggravation after seeming for a short time to have improved (pars. 58 to 62 and par. 69).

24

Therefore, none but the homoeopathic method of applying remedies to diseases promises to be helpful.

This therapy chooses from among all the remedies whose actions upon the healthy have been established that one which has the power and propensity to produce an artificial disease condition most similar to the natural one being treated. This remedy is used for the totality of symptoms of a case after the exciting cause, where known, and any additional circumstances have been considered.

25

Pure experiment[a]—the only infallible guide in the art of healing—teaches us in all tests conscientiously conducted that the medicine that has produced upon a healthy human body the greatest number of symptoms *similar* to those of the disease being treated is the only one that will cure. Administered properly potentized, in small doses, this medicine will rapidly, thoroughly, and permanently destroy the totality of the symptoms of the disease, which means the whole disease itself, changing it into health (par. 6 to par. 16).

All medicines without exception cure those diseases whose symptoms most closely resemble their own, and leave none of them uncured.

a. I am not referring here to the kind of experiment of which the usual physician of the old school boasts. After treating for years with polypharmaceutic prescriptions a number of diseases that they have never properly examined but recognize only according to the categories of orthodox pathology, they fancy that they see in them an imaginary disease substance or some other hypothetical inner abnormality.

They always see something, but never know what it is; they obtain results that no human but only a god could decipher in such a muddle of forces converging on an unknown object, results from which there is nothing to be learned, nothing to be gained. Fifty years of this sort of experimentation are like fifty years spent looking into a kaleidoscope fitted with multicolored unknown things endlessly revolving upon themselves: in the end one has seen thousands of shapes perpetually changing, without accounting for any of them.

26

This is in accordance with the natural law of homoeopathy, which has always been the basis of all true cure, a law sometimes anticipated in the past, certainly, but never acknowledged before now:

In the living organism a weaker dynamic affection is permanently extinguished by a stronger one, which, though different in nature, nevertheless greatly resembles it in expression.[a]

a. Both physical and moral disturbances are cured in this way.

Why does brilliant Jupiter disappear in the light of dawn to the optic nerve of the beholder? Because a very similar though greater power, the light of dawning day, acts upon the optic nerve. How does one effectively calm olfactory nerves offended by disagreeable odors? By snuff, which affects the smell similarly but more strongly. Neither with music nor with sweets could we cure this disgust of smells, because they act upon different sensory nerves. By what device did the clever soldier drown in the compassionate ears of onlookers the whimpering of those who ran the gauntlet? By the shrill, exhilarating sound of the high-pitched fife, coupled with the noisy drum. And how did he cover the distant thunder of enemy cannons, which struck terror in his army? By the deep, quaking rumble of the big drum. He could not have obtained these results by reprimanding the regiment or by distributing bright uniforms!

In the same way sorrow and mourning are extinguished in the soul at the news, albeit fictitious, that a greater misfortune has befallen someone else; the negative effects of intense joy are removed by coffee, which in itself produces a state of excessive joyfulness.

A people like the Germans, gradually sinking for centuries ever deeper into an attitude of obsequious slavery and abject apathy, had to be trodden into the dust still more deeply and to the very limit of endurance by the western conqueror before their self-contempt exceeded itself to the point of being overcome and the feeling of their human dignity returned, so that at last they raised their heads again as Germans.

27

The curative virtue of medicines thus depends on their symptoms being similar to those of the disease, but stronger (par. 12 to par. 26).

It follows that in any particular case, a disease can be destroyed and removed most surely, thoroughly, swiftly, and permanently only by a medicine that can make a human being feel a totality of symptoms most completely similar to it but stronger.

28

Since this natural law of healing is confirmed in all objective experiments and authentic experience in the world, it is established as a fact. Scientific explanations of *how it works* are of little importance, and I see little value in attempting one. Nevertheless, the one that follows proves itself the most likely, because it is founded on experience.

29

Any disease that is not exclusively a surgical case consists of a particular pathological, dynamic untunement of feelings and functions in our vital force (vital principle).

So in homoeopathic cure this vital principle, which has been dynamically untuned by natural disease, is *taken over* by a similar and somewhat stronger artificial disease, through the administration of a potentized medicine that has been accurately chosen for the similarity of its symptoms.

Consequently the (weaker) natural dynamic disease is extinguished and disappears; from then on it no longer exists for the vital principle, which is controlled and occupied only by the stronger artificial disease; this in turn presently wanes, so that the patient is left free and cured.[a] Thus delivered, the *dynamis* can again maintain the organism in health.

This explanation, the most likely one, is based on the propositions following.

a. The vital force frees itself much more easily from artificial diseases than from natural ones, although the former are stronger, because the disease agents called medicines producing the artificial diseases have a short action.

Natural diseases (of psoric, syphilitic, and sycotic nature), though weaker than artificial ones, have a longer action, nearly always as long as life itself, and cannot be overcome and extinguished by the vital force without the help of a therapeutic agent. To extinguish them the physician acts on the vital force with a power (the homoeopathic remedy) that can make a very similar but stronger artificial disease. A disease of many years' duration (par. 46) being cured by an outbreak of smallpox or measles—both of these running their course in a few weeks—is a similar occurrence.

30

Because the right medicines cure and overcome natural diseases, it would seem that the human organism is altered more surely by medicines than by natural disease agents (especially since we can control the dosage of the medicines).

31

The psychic and physical inimical influences that we encounter in the world and that we call disease agents do not have an absolute power to untune our organism.[a] We fall ill under their influence only when the organism is disposed and susceptible enough to their attack for its feelings and functions to be altered and untuned from the normal. Thus these disease agents do not make everybody sick each time.

a. When I speak of disease as a tuning or untuning of the human economy, far be it from me to attempt a metaphysical explanation of the inner nature of disease in general or of any particular case of disease. I am merely pointing out that diseases obviously *are not* and *cannot be* mechanical or chemical changes in the material substance of the body, that they do not depend on a material disease substance, but are an exclusively dynamic, spirit-like untunement of life.

32

But artificial pathogenetic forces that we call medicines are quite a different matter.

Every real medicine can at *all* times and in *all* circumstances affect *every* living person and bring about its particular symptoms in him (even clearly perceptible ones if the dose is large enough). It follows that every living human organism can at all times and without exception (*unconditionally*) be affected—as it were, infected—by a medicinal disease; and, as I have said, this is not at all the case with natural diseases.

33

From all experience it therefore follows incontrovertibly that the living human organism is far more susceptible to and disposed to be influenced by medicinal pathogenetic forces than by ordinary natural ones and contagious miasms.[a] In other words, *natural disease agents have only a subordinate and conditional, often very conditional, power to alter human health, while medicinal forces have a far superior power to do so, one that is absolute and unconditional.*

a. A striking example of this: Until 1801, epidemics of Sydenham's smooth scarlatina broke out from time to time among children and attacked without exception all those who had not yet been exposed. But in the *Königslutter* epidemic, which I witnessed, *all* the children who had taken a very small dose of *Belladonna* early enough remained immune to this very infectious disease.

If medicines can protect us from the contagion of a raging epidemic, they must possess a greater power to alter our vital force than the epidemic.

34

However, the artificial disease brought on by a medicine does not have only to be stronger in order to cure the natural disease.

Above all it must have the greatest possible similarity to the natural disease being treated. By its somewhat greater strength it has to transform the disturbance of the vital principle, which is instinctive, unreasoning, and without memory, into an artificial disease condition very similar to the natural one. It must not just dim the vital principle's sensation of the natural disease condition but extinguish it completely and destroy it.

This is so true that nature itself cannot cure even a somewhat old disease by adding a new dissimilar one, however strong. Nor can medical treatment bring this about, as the allopaths try to do, with medicines that do *not* have the ability to produce in a healthy individual a disease state *similar* to the one being treated.

35

To illustrate this we shall consider the three different possibilities that may occur when two dissimilar diseases meet in the same person, whether they are two dissimilar natural diseases, or

a natural disease and a medicinal disease that are
dissimilar, the latter resulting from the common
and inappropriate allopathic treatment with medicines that cannot cause an artificial disease
condition similar to the one being treated.

From this we shall prove, on the one hand, that not
even nature can cure an existing disease with a new
dissimilar unhomoeopathic one even if it is stronger
and, on the other, that medicines, however powerful,
will never truly cure any disease if they are used un-
homoeopathically.

36

I. Two *dissimilar* natural diseases (one pre-existing
the other) meeting in the same patient: If they are
equally strong or *if the first is stronger* than the second,
the more recent is repelled.

Thus someone suffering from a grave chronic disease
will not be affected by autumn dysentery or by any
other mild epidemic.

According to Larrey, the Levant plague does not
break out in places where scurvy is prevalent, and
people suffering from tetter are not infected either.[a]

Jenner holds that in people who have rickets, smallpox vaccination does not take.

Von Hildenbrand asserts that people with phthisis do
not catch mild epidemic fevers.

a. Larrey, "Mémoires et observations," in *Dé-
scription de l'Egypte,* vol. I.

37

In the same way, old chronic diseases remain uncured and unchanged from the *usual allopathic treatment,* i.e., treatment with remedies that cannot produce in healthy individuals a condition similar to any part of the disease.

They do not respond to such treatment even when it is prolonged for years if these treatments are mild.[a] This is verified in practice daily and needs no further corroboration.

    a. On the other hand, if the disease is treated with violent allopathic drugs, other graver, more life-threatening ailments are created in its place.

38

II. *If the later dissimilar disease is the stronger,* it temporarily suppresses and suspends the former milder one, until the new disease has run its course or been cured; then the old affection reappears, *uncured.*

Two epileptic children who contracted *tinea capitis* stopped having epileptic seizures, but these reappeared unchanged as soon as the eruption on the head went away, according to Nicolaas Tulp.[a]

Schoepf observed the disappearance of scabies as soon as scurvy appeared and its return as soon as the scurvy was cured.[b]

A violent infection of typhus interrupted the progress of phthisis, which continued to evolve as soon as the typhus ended.[c]

When mania comes on in a patient with phthisis, it suspends this disease with all its symptoms, but the phthisis comes back and pursues its course to fatal termination immediately after the mental disturbance ceases.[d]

When measles and smallpox occur simultaneously in the same child, the measles, which manifest earlier, are usually stopped by the smallpox, which manifests later; the measles reappear and resume their development only after the smallpox is completely gone. The opposite also happens not infrequently: Manget observes that inoculated smallpox is not infrequently suspended for four days if measles appear at this time, and it resumes its development to the end after the desquamation of the measles.[e] John Hunter says that an infection of measles arrested the inflammation of a smallpox vaccination six days after the inoculation had taken and that the pustules broke out only after the measles had run their seven-day course.[f]

During a measles epidemic the measles eruption came on in a number of patients the fourth or the fifth day after smallpox inoculation and during its entire course prevented the smallpox pustules from forming; they developed and ran their course only after this period.[g]

Sydenham's true, smooth, erysipelas-like scarlet fever, with sore throat, was interrupted the fourth day by cowpox, which continued its development to the end, after which the scarlet fever returned.[h] But since these two diseases seem equally strong, it has also happened that the cowpox was interrupted on the eighth day by the beginning of a case of Sydenham's true, smooth scarlet fever. The red cowpox areola disappeared until the scarlet fever was over, when it returned and continued to the end.[i]

A case of cowpox was suspended suddenly near its climax on the eighth day by the appearance of measles. After the desquamation of the latter, the cowpox resumed its development in such a way that, according to Kortum, it appeared on the sixteenth day as it normally would have appeared on the tenth.[j] The same writer saw cowpox inoculation take during a case of measles contracted earlier, but its development was postponed until the measles were over.[k]

I myself saw mumps (angina parotidea) disappear as soon as a cowpox inoculation had taken and approached its climax. Only after the pustules and their red areola had disappeared did the feverish swelling of the parotoid and submaxillary glands, caused by the mumps miasm, come back and run its seven-day course.

This is the case with all dissimilar diseases; the stronger suspends the weaker (unless they complicate each other, which rarely happens in acute affections). But never do they cure each other.

a. Obs., lib. I, obs. 8.

b. In Hufeland's *Journal,* vol. XV, p. 2.

c. Chevalier, in Hufeland's *Neuesten Annalen der französischen Heilkunde,* vol. II, p. 192.

d. Reil, *Memorab.,* fasc. III, p. 171. *Mania phtisi superveniens eam cum omnibus suis phaenomenis aufert, verum mox redit phthisis et occidit abeunta mania.* ["The mania of a consumptive person, coming upon him, removes it (the illness) with all of its symptoms, but presently the illness of the consumptive returns and destroys him if the mania is discontinued."]

e. In *Edinb. Med. Comment.,* vol. I. p. 1.

f. John Hunter, *On the Venereal Diseases,* p. 5.

g. Rainay, in *Edinb. Med. Comment.,* vol. III, p. 480.

h. Also described very accurately by Withering and Plenciz. It is entirely different from *purpura miliaris* fever (or Roodvonk fever), which was also, incorrectly, called scarlet fever. Only in recent years have these two diseases, originally very different, begun to resemble each other in their symptoms.

i. Jenner, in *Medicinische Annalen,* August 1800, p. 747.

j. In Hufeland's *Journal der praktischen Arznei-kunde,* vol. XX, no. 3, p. 50.

k. Loc. cit.

39

The orthodox school has witnessed for centuries that nature itself has never once cured any existing disease with another *dissimilar* one, however intense.

What must we think of this school, which nevertheless has continued to treat chronic diseases allopathically, with medicines and formulas that can only cause a disease condition—God knows which—*dissimilar* to the one being treated? Even if these physicians have not hitherto observed nature attentively enough, the miserable results of their treatment should have taught them that they were on the wrong road. Haven't they seen that their usual practice of employing violent allopathic means to treat chronic disease only creates a *dissimilar* artificial disease, which, as long as it is maintained, merely silences, suppresses, and suspends the original trouble? Haven't they seen that the original disease reappears, and always has to reappear, as soon as the decline of the patient's strength no longer permits the allopathic attack on his life to continue?

In this way, of course, by violent and frequently repeated purgatives, a scabies eruption will disappear quite quickly from the skin. But when the patient can no longer tolerate the *dissimilar* intestinal disease inflicted on him by the purges and has to stop taking them, either the skin eruption breaks out as before or else the internal psora develops some grave symptom, since, in addition to his original trouble, which remains undiminished, the patient now suffers a painfully ruined digestion and the exhaustion brought on by purging.

Thus when orthodox physicians bring about artificial skin ulcers and sustain fontanels on the exterior of the body in an effort to remove a chronic disease, they can *never* reach their objective, they can *never* heal the chronic disease, because such artificial skin ulcers are completely foreign and allopathic to the internal disease. Since, however, the irritation of the multiple fontanels constitutes a *dissimilar* disease at least sometimes stronger than the indwelling one, it initially silences and suspends it, but *only* for a very short period, sometimes for a couple of weeks, while the patient gradually wastes away. As Pechlin[a] and others have stated, epilepsy suppressed for many years by fontanels always returns worse than ever as soon as the fontanels are allowed to heal. The fontanels are not more foreign, dissimilar, and violently allopathic to the epilepsy, nor the purges to the scabies, than all those mixtures of unknown ingredients used in common practice are to all the other innumerable known and unknown forms of disease that they treat. These mixtures merely moderate, suppress, and suspend the trouble without curing it, and only for a short time, and their prolonged use always adds a new disease condition to the old one.

a. *Obs. phys. med.,* lib. 2, obs. 30.

40

III. It can also happen that the *new disease,* after acting for a long time on the organism, finally joins the *old one, dissimilar to it,* forming with it a *complex disease.* Each occupies a particular region of the organism, only, as it were, the site characteristically belonging to it—i.e., the organs with which it has a special affinity—and abandons the rest to the disease that is dissimilar to it.

Thus a patient with venereal disease can still contract scabies and vice versa; *but these two diseases, being dissimilar, cannot extinguish or cure each other.* At the beginning, while the scabies eruption is starting to appear, the venereal symptoms diminish and are suspended; but in time (since the venereal disease is at least as strong as the scabies) the two become associated,[a] i.e., each takes over only the particular parts of the organism with which it has an affinity, and the patient thereby becomes more ill and more difficult to cure.

When two dissimilar acute contagious diseases meet—e.g., smallpox and measles—as I have said, one usually suspends the other. Nevertheless, there have been rare instances in violent epidemics when two dissimilar acute diseases have appeared in one and the same body and, as it were, complicated each other for a short time.

During simultaneous epidemics of smallpox and measles, P. Russel found only one case in which the eruptions of these two dissimilar diseases appeared in the same person at the same time.[b] Among those affected there were 300 cases in which the two diseases excluded or suspended each other until the first disease had completely run its course; in a certain number the measles, initially suspended, only erupted twenty days after the smallpox eruption; in others the smallpox erupted seventeen to eighteen days after the measles eruption.

Rainay saw in two girls smallpox and measles existing together.[c] J. Maurice said that he had observed only two such cases in his entire practice.[d]

One encounters similar examples in Ettmüller[e] and a few others.

Zencker saw cowpox follow its regular course along with measles and along with miliary fever,[f] and Jenner saw cowpox follow its course undisturbed during a mercury treatment for syphilis.

a. Precise experiments and cures obtained in this category of complex diseases have by now completely convinced me that they are not a fusion but instead that in such cases the two dissimilar diseases exist only *beside* each other in the organism, each in the parts for which it has an affinity, since their cure is completely accomplished by the timely alternation of the best antisyphilitic and antiscabies remedies, each prepared in the most appropriate way and administered in the most appropriate dose.

b. V. *Transactions of a Society for the Improvement of Med. and Chir. Knowledge,* vol. II.

c. In *Edinb. Med. Comment.,* vol. III, p. 480.

d. In *Med. and Phys. Journ.,* 1805.

e. Opera, vol. II, pt. I, chap. 10.

f. In Hufeland's *Journal,* vol. XVII.

41

The association and mutual complication of dissimilar natural diseases in the same body occur much less frequently than those disease complications that are the usual result of inappropriate allopathic treatment through *the prolonged use of unsuitable medicines.*

From the continual repetition of unsuitable medicines, new and often very chronic disease conditions corresponding to the nature of these drugs associate themselves with the natural disease being treated. These medicinal disease conditions cannot cure the natural disease, because the substances used do not act upon it by similarity of effect, i.e., homoeopathically. Gradually they combine with the dissimilar chronic trouble, complicating it, so that a new dissimilar artificial disease of chronic nature is added to the old one. Thus the patient who was simply ill is now doubly so, so much more ill and difficult to cure that he sometimes becomes incurable, often even dies. Many cases discussed in medical journals and reported in the literature attest to the truth of this.

Similar are the frequent cases in which syphilis that has been complicated, especially with scabies but also with chronic fig-wart gonorrhea, far from being cured by prolonged or frequently repeated treatment with large doses of inappropriate mercury preparations, takes a place in the organism next to the chronic mercury disease that the medicine has gradually engendered.[a]

This forms a complex disease, often quite monstrous, generally called masked venereal disease, which, if it is not completely incurable, can nevertheless be cured only with the greatest difficulty.

a. Mercury administered in large doses engenders new diseases and causes considerable destruction in the organism, especially when the venereal disease is complicated with psora, which is frequently the case, since, besides symptoms similar to those of syphilis, by which it can cure syphilis homoeopathically, mercury has in its nature many others that are dissimilar to it, e.g., exostoses and caries of the bones, etc.

42

As we have seen in paragraph 40, nature sometimes allows in certain cases the coexistence of two (even three) natural diseases in one and the same body. But we should note that this complication takes place only with *dissimilar* diseases: according to eternal laws of nature, they cannot eliminate, destroy, or cure each other.

This entanglement seems to take place in such a way that the two (or the three) diseases divide the organism among themselves, each occupying the organs and systems with which it has a characteristic affinity. Because of the dissimilarity of these diseases to each other, this division can take place without denying the unity of life.

43

But the result is quite different when two *similar* diseases meet the organism, i.e., when a similar and stronger disease is added to the one already there. Here we observe the way in which cure can take place in nature and the way in which men should cure.

44

Two *similar* diseases can neither *ward off* each other (sec. I, par. 36, par. 37) nor *suspend* each other (sec. II, par. 38, par. 39) in such a way that the older of the two comes back after the disappearance of the more recent. Nor can two *similar* diseases *exist next to each other* (sec. III, par. 40, par. 41) in the same organism and form a complex of *two* diseases.

45

No! Two diseases, different in nature[a] but very similar in their manifestations and effects, their respective suffering and symptoms, always and infallibly destroy each other as soon as they meet in the organism. It is not difficult to understand why the stronger destroys the weaker: it has a similar action, and because of its *predominance,* takes over precisely *those parts of the organism until then affected by the weaker one,* which since it can now no longer act, disappears.[b]

In other words, as soon as the new disease agent, similar to the first but stronger, takes over the patient's sensations, the vital principle, because of its unity, can no longer feel the weaker similar one; it is extinguished, it exists no more, since it is never something material but only a dynamic (spirit-like) affection. The vital principle therefore remains affected (but only fleetingly) exclusively by the new similar but stronger disease force of the medicine.

a. See footnote to paragraph 26.

b. Just as the image of a lamp flame on the optic nerve is quickly overcome and wiped out by the stronger sunbeam falling on the eye.

46

We could cite very many examples of homoeopathic cures brought about by natural diseases with similar symptoms. But since we require precise and indubitable data we shall confine ourselves to the small number, always true to type, arising from unvarying miasms, which give them a distinct name.

Smallpox, prominent among them and so notorious for its many violent symptoms, has removed and cured a host of ills that have similar symptoms.

How common are the ophthalmias of smallpox and how violent, even to blindness! Through inoculation smallpox completely and permanently cured chronic eye inflammation in a case cited by Dezoteux[a] and in another cited by Leroy.[b]

A person who was blind for two years after the suppression of a scalp eruption completely recovered his sight after smallpox, according to Klein.[c]

How often has smallpox not brought about deafness and dyspnea! And it removed both these chronic complaints when it reached its acme, as J. F. Closs observes.[d]

Swelling of the testicles, even very severe, is a frequent symptom of smallpox; and that is why it could, by similarity, cure a large, hard swelling of the left testicle caused by a trauma (Klein).[e] Another observer also notes that it cured a similar testicular swelling.[f]

Among the unpleasant complaints that occur in smallpox there is a particular dysentery-like stool; and so, by similarity, smallpox has cured dysentery (F. Wendt).[g]

It is well known that smallpox contracted during cowpox immediately wipes out the cowpox homoeopathically and aborts it, both because of its greater strength and because of its close similarity. On the other hand, if the cowpox is already near maturity, because of its great similarity to the supervening smallpox, the latter is at least greatly attenuated homoeopathically,[h] and milder, as Mühry[i] and many others have stated.

In the lymph of the cowpox inoculation there is, in addition to the element that protects against smallpox, a quite different substance that causes an overall skin eruption usually of small, dry (sometimes rather large, suppurating) pimples surrounded by a red areola and often intermixed with round red spots, often itching most violently.

In many children this eruption comes out several days *before* the red cowpox areola appears; but more often it comes out several days *afterward* and disappears in a couple of days, leaving behind small, hard, red spots. It is through their similarity to this secondary infectious agent that skin eruptions of children, often very old and troublesome ones, are homoeopathically cured, completely and permanently, by the cowpox vaccination as soon as it takes, something many observers have noticed.[j]

Cowpox, which has a characteristic swelling of the arm among its symptoms,[k] cured a swollen, half-paralyzed arm after breaking out.[l]

The fever that comes in cowpox with the appearance of the red areola has cured (homoeopathically) two cases of intermittent fever, as Hardege the Younger reports.[m] This confirms J. Hunter's remark that two fevers (similar diseases) cannot exist in the same body at the same time.[n]

There is much similarity between the fevers and coughs of measles and those of whooping cough. In an epidemic where these two diseases raged simultaneously, Bosquillon noticed that many children who had just had measles remained free from whooping cough.[o] They would all have remained permanently free of whooping cough and would have been rendered immune by the measles if whooping cough were not just partly similar to measles, i.e., if it also had a similar skin eruption. That is why measles protected only a number of children from the whooping cough, and only during that epidemic.

But when measles meets a disease that is similar to it in its main symptom—the eruption—it will undeniably destroy and cure it homoeopathically.

Thus a chronic herpetic eruption was cured[p] (homoeopathically) promptly, completely, and permanently by an eruption of measles, as Kortum observes.[q]

A six-year-old miliary eruption on the throat, face, and arms, with extreme burning, which was aggravated whenever the weather changed, was reduced to a simple swelling of the skin when measles broke out; and after the measles it was cured, never to return.[r]

a. Traité de l'inoculation, p. 189.

b. Heilkunde für Mütter, p. 384.

c. Interpres clinicus, p. 293.

d. Neue Heilart der Kinderpocken, Ulm, 1769, p. 68; and *Specim.*, obs. 18.

e. Op. cit.

f. Nov. Act. Nat. Cur., vol. I, obs. 22.

g. Nachricht von dem Krankeninstitut zu Erlangen, 1783.

h. This seems to be the reason for the remarkable

salutary result of the widespread use of Jenner's cow-pox vaccination. The smallpox has not since then appeared among us with such widespread virulence. Forty or fifty years ago, when a city was stricken, it lost at least half, often three-quarters of its children.

i. Willan, *Ueber die Kuhpockenimpfung.*

j. Especially Clavier, Hurel, and Desormeaux, in *Bulletin des sciences médicales, publié par les membres du comité central de la Société de Médecine du Département de l'Eure,* 1808; also in *Journal de médecine continué,* vol. XV, p. 206.

k. Balhorn, in Hufeland's *Journal,* vol. X, p. 2.

l. Stevenson, in Duncan's *Annals of Medicine,* lustr. II, vol. I, pt. II, no. 9.

m. In Hufeland's *Journal,* vol. XXIII.

n. On the Venereal Diseases, p. 4.

o. Cullen's *Eléments de médecine pratique,* French translation, pt. II, I, 3, chap. 7.

p. Or at least that symptom was removed.

q. In Hufeland's *Journal,* vol. XX, no. 3, p. 50.

r. Rau, *Ueber d. Werth des hom. Heilv.,* Heidelberg, 1824, p. 85.

47

It would be impossible to find clearer, more convincing examples than these to teach a physician the best way of choosing artificial disease agents (medicines) to cure surely, rapidly, permanently, according to natural law.

48

All the examples we have mentioned show us that neither nature nor the physician's art can destroy and cure an ailment or a disease with a dissimilar disease agent, however strong, but only with one that can produce *similar symptoms* and is *slightly stronger,* according to eternal and irrevocable laws of nature hitherto not recognized.

49

We would find far more such authentic natural homoeopathic cures if, on the one hand, observers had been more attentive to them and if, on the other hand, nature were not so poor in remedial homoeopathic diseases.

50

As instruments of homoeopathic cure we see that powerful nature itself has hardly more than the few fixed miasmatic diseases—scabies, measles, and smallpox.[a] But some of these disease agents are more mortally dangerous and more to be feared as remedies than the diseases that they treat,[b] and some, after curing similar diseases, have in turn to be cured (e.g., scabies). Both these circumstances make their use as homoeopathic remedies difficult, uncertain, and dangerous.

Besides, how few disease conditions there are among men which find their similar (homoeopathic) remedy in smallpox, measles, and scabies! That is why nature can cure only very few diseases through such perilous homoeopathic means.

Such processes are all the more fraught with danger and serious drawbacks because, unlike medicines, their dosage cannot be reduced to fit the circumstances. Quite the contrary: in order to be cured of an old disease the patient is afflicted with all the troublesome and dangerous suffering of the whole, new, similar disease of smallpox, measles, or scabies.

Nevertheless, we can point to beautiful homoeopathic cures from the fortunate encounter of similar diseases, so many eloquent proofs of the one great natural law of healing which rules in them: *Cure by means of symptom similarity.*

a. And the above-mentioned exanthematous agent existing in the cowpox lymph.

b. Viz., smallpox and measles.

51

Such occurrences are enough to reveal conclusively to our intelligence this law of healing. But see what advantage man has over the chance happenings of crude nature! Does he not have in the medicinal substances distributed throughout creation so many more thousands of homoeopathic curative agents with which to help his suffering brothers! They give him the means of creating all possible variations of disease conditions with which to treat innumerable conceivable and inconceivable natural diseases homoeopathically.

Once they have achieved their curative purpose, the action of these medicinal disease agents disappears by itself and is overcome by the vital force without having to be expelled in its turn, like scabies.

The physician can dilute, subdivide, and potentize these artificial disease agents almost infinitely, thereby reducing their dosage until they are only slightly stronger than the similar natural diseases they treat.

Thus in this incomparable therapy there is no need to attack the organism with violence in order to destroy an inveterate ailment. The suffering and torment of natural disease give way to the desired state of permanent health gently, imperceptibly, and often quite rapidly.

52

There are only two principal therapies:

the first, based in every respect exclusively on the exact observation of nature, and on scrupulous experiments and pure experience—the *homoeopathic method, never* wittingly used before me, and

the second, which does not do this: the *allopathic*
(or *heteropathic*) *method*.

They are directly opposed to each other, and only
someone *who does not know either* could be fool
enough to suppose that they could ever approach each
other or unite, could make himself so ridiculous as to
treat homoeopathically one moment and allopathically
the next to please his patients. This is a criminal be-
trayal of divine homoeopathy!

53

True, gentle cures are exclusively homoeopathic.
This method, as we have found above in a different
manner, through conclusions derived from experience
(par. 7 to par. 25), is incontrovertibly the correct way of
achieving the most certain, most rapid, most permanent
cure of diseases, because it is based on an eternal and
infallible law of nature.

The *pure homoeopathic* method of healing is the
only correct one, the only one possible to human art;
it is the most direct one, just as certainly as there is
but one possible straight line between two given
points.

54

The *allopathic* method, which has tried so many different things against diseases, but of course always inappropriate ones (ἀλλοῖα), has been the dominant therapy from the beginning of human memory and has expressed itself in widely varying forms called systems. In
time each of these systems was followed by another
completely different one, yet each had the honor of being called *rational medicine*.[a]

Each of the founders of these systems pretentiously

claimed that he could penetrate and understand the intimate essence of human life in health and in disease. Accordingly he decreed *which materia peccans*[b] should be removed from the patient and *how* it should be done to cure him, all this according to vain suppositions and pet assumptions, without sincerely questioning nature and impartially heeding experience.

They held that diseases were conditions that always manifested themselves in rather the same way. That is why most of these systems gave names to their fictitious disease images, each classifying them differently. They attributed to remedies on conjecture (see all the different materiae medicae!) actions that were supposed to remove these abnormal conditions—i.e., cure them.[c]

a. As if a science that should be based only on the observation of natural phenomena and experiment could be arrived at by idle speculation and scholastic arguments!

b. Because until very recently people looked for that which had to be cured in diseases in a *material* to be expelled, since they could not rise to the conception of a dynamic (footnote, par. 11) action of disease forces and medicines in the life of the animal organism.

c. To crown their self-delusion, they mixed (very learnedly) more than one, indeed, several different drugs in their so-called prescriptions and administered them in frequent large doses. Thus precious and fragile human life, so easily destroyed, was frequently placed in jeopardy at the hands of these perverted people, especially since bleedings, emetics, purges, blistering plaster, fontanels, setons, caustics, and cauterizations were also used.

55

Shortly after each of these systems and therapies was introduced, it became clear to the public that by following any of them exactly the suffering of patients was only increased and multiplied, and one would long since have abandoned these allopathic doctors completely but for the fact that they managed somewhat to maintain their credibility by providing *palliative relief* to patients from time to time with a few empirically discovered remedies that were spectacular for their flattering, often almost instantaneous action.

56

With this *palliative (antipathic, enantiopathic) method,* introduced seventeen centuries ago, following the teaching of Galen, *contraria contrariis,* physicians could until today hope to win the patient's trust most infallibly by deceiving him with almost instantaneous improvement. From the following we shall see just how fundamentally unhelpful, how harmful this type of treatment is (in diseases that do not pass quickly).

In fact, this is the only thing in allopathic therapy that has any evident relationship to a portion of the symptomatology of the natural disease—but what relationship? In truth the opposite of the right one; it should be scrupulously avoided if one does not wish to deceive and mock the chronically ill.[a]

a. There are those who would like to introduce a third kind of therapy, called *isopathy,* treating a disease with the identical miasm that produced it. But if this were possible, since this miasm would reach the patient only in highly potentized and therefore altered form, it would cure by opposing a *simillimum* to the *simillimo. To try to cure* in this way, with an exactly identical *disease agent* (*per idem*), runs counter to all common sense and therefore also to all experience.

Those who first introduced this so-called isopathy probably had in mind the good that had been done to humanity by vaccination: those who were vaccinated remained free from all future smallpox contagion and were cured of the disease in advance, as it were.

Cowpox and smallpox are only very similar, however, and not the same disease at all; they differ in many respects, especially in the quicker development and the mildness of cowpox, but above all in the fact that it is never contracted by man through proximity. The widespread use of vaccination has so effectively put an end to all epidemics of the terribly deadly smallpox that the present generation no longer has any clear idea of this hideous bygone scourge. Other diseases peculiar to animals can of course also be used as medicines to cure *very similar* and important human diseases, happily increasing the number of homoeopathic remedies available.

But trying to cure with a human disease substance—for instance, using a psoricum derived from human scabies to treat that same disease in man, or troubles arising from it—is going too far! Nothing can come of it but misfortune and aggravation of the disease.

57

The orthodox physician who treats according to this antipathic method gives a remedy for a single troublesome symptom, disregarding all the rest, a remedy that is known to bring out the exact opposite of the symptom to be subdued and that can be expected to produce the speediest (palliative) relief; age-old medicine has instructed him to do this for more than fifteen hundred years: *contraria contrariis.*

He gives strong doses of opium for pains of all sorts because it quickly benumbs all sensations; he even gives it for diarrhea, because it quickly inhibits peristaltic action of the intestines and anesthetizes them, and for insomnia, because it speedily induces a stupefying, comatose sleep. He gives purgatives for inveterate constipation; he immerses the burned hand in cold water, and the coldness seems instantaneously and magically to take away the pain of the burn; he puts the chilly patient into warm baths, which warm him up, but only for a moment; he gives wine to someone who is chronically weakened, which revives and quickens him for a moment. There are other antipathic remedial measures that he uses as well, but only a few, because orthodox medicine knows the characteristic primary action of but a small number of medicines.

58

In judging this method of using drugs I shall overlook for now its *fundamental error* of prescribing *only symptomatically* (see footnote to par. 7)—i.e., narrowly, *for only one of the symptoms,* only a small part of the whole, therefore obviously without relieving the totality of the disease, which is the only thing the patient can want.

But let us question experience: Among all the cases in which medicines were used antipathically for chronic or persistent complaints, is there one in which temporary relief was not followed by the aggravation not only of the symptom at first palliated but indeed of the whole disease?

Every conscientious observer will agree that after this

short antipathic amelioration, aggravation follows *in every case without exception,* even though the orthodox physician usually explains this aggravation to the patient differently, blaming it on the malignity, only now revealed, of the original disease or on the appearance of some new disease.[a]

 a. No matter how little physicians have hitherto been wont to observe, the aggravation inevitably following upon such palliation could not have escaped them. We find a striking example of this in J. H. Schulze's *Diss. qua corporis humani momentanearum alterationum specimina quaedam expenduntur* [Dissertation on how certain indications of momentary changes in the human body are reckoned], Halae, 1741, par. 28. Willis reports something similar in *Pharm. rat.,* sec. 7, chap. 1, p. 298: *Opiata dolores atrocissimos plerumque sedant atque indolentiam procurant, eamque aliquamdiu et pro stato quodam tempore continuant, quo spatio elapso, dolores mox recrudescunt et brevi ad solitam ferociam augentur.* ["Opiates generally assuage the most severe pains and produce insensibility, and they continue the insensibility for a while, even for a fixed time. When that space of time has passed, the pains soon return and in a short time are increased to their accustomed degree of severity."] And also on p. 295: *Exactis opii viribus illico redeunt tormina, nec atrocitatem suam remittunt, nisi dum ab eodem pharmaco rursus incantatur.* ["When the strength of the opium has been spent, immediately the gripes return, nor do they slacken their severity unless they are enchanted away again by the same drug."] J. Hunter (*On the Venereal Diseases,* p. 13) said that wine increases the energy of weak people without imparting to them any real strength and that their spirits afterward decline as much as they were at first stimulated, so that they gain nothing but, on the contrary, usually lose much of their strength.

59

The salient symptoms of a long-standing disease have *never* in this world been treated in this palliative, antipathic way without reappearing in a few hours, often manifestly worse.

To overcome a chronic tendency toward daytime drowsiness, coffee is prescribed. Its primary action is to stimulate, but when it no longer has any effect, the daytime drowsiness increases.

For frequent waking at night opium is prescribed before retiring, without consideration of the other symptoms of the disease. Because of its primary action it procures a stupefying, comatose sleep for one night, but the following nights are even more sleepless.

This same opium is used for chronic diarrheas without consideration of the other symptoms; its primary action constipates, but after being checked briefly, the diarrhea returns worse than before.

Severe, frequently recurring pains of all kinds can be suppressed with opium, which deadens feeling, but only for a short time; the pains always return worse than before, often to the point of being intolerable, or else are replaced by other, far worse troubles.

For inveterate nocturnal cough the ordinary physician knows of nothing better than to give opium, which in its primary action suppresses all irritation. The cough will perhaps disappear the first night, but it returns all the more intensely on the following nights, and if the physician continues to suppress it with increasingly strong doses of this palliative, fever and night sweats are added to the disturbance.

For weakness of the bladder and the pitiful retention of urine resulting, cantharides tincture is used to stimulate the urinary passages antipathically, and although this does at first force the evacuation of urine, the bladder subsequently becomes less capable of being stimulated and contracting, until paralysis is imminent.

A chronic tendency to constipation is said to yield to strong doses of purgatives and laxative salts. They do irritate the bowels to frequent evacuation, but their secondary action constipates still further.

The ordinary physician tries to overcome chronic weakness by prescribing the drinking of wine, but only its primary action stimulates; in its consequent secondary effect, the patient's forces sink that much more.

He maintains that bitter things and hot spices strengthen and warm a chronically weak and cold stomach. Only the primary action of these palliatives stimulates the stomach, and their secondary action makes it all the more inactive.

Chilliness and a chronic lack of vital heat are supposed to respond to warm baths, but afterward the patients are weaker and more chilly than before.

Cold water does bring immediate relief to the pain of a severe burn, but afterward the pain increases incredibly, as inflammation spreads to the surrounding tissues and increases.

The allopaths treat chronic stoppage of the nose from coryza with remedies that cause sneezing and the secretion of mucus, but they fail to observe that this antipathic treatment progressively aggravates the condition in its secondary action, so that the nose is blocked even more than before.

The primary action of electricity and galvanism powerfully stimulates muscular movement and immediately produces energetic motion in chronically weak, almost paralyzed limbs, but its secondary action is the complete deadening of all muscular irritability and complete paralysis.

Bloodletting is held to remove chronic congestion of the head and other parts—e.g., where there is palpitation—but it is always followed by greater congestion in these organs, stronger, more rapid palpitations, etc.

Ordinary medicine knows of no better way to treat the paralytic torpor of body and mind coupled with unconsciousness found in many kinds of typhus than with strong doses of valerian, because it is one of the most powerful stimulants known. But in their ignorance these physicians are unaware that this is only the primary action of the drug and that in the secondary action (counteraction) that follows, the organism unfailingly relapses into even greater torpor and immobility, that is, into paralysis of the mental and bodily organs, even death. They do not see that precisely those patients to whom they have fed the most valerian (used antipathically) are the ones most certain to die.

The physician of the old school[a] rejoices when he has forcibly slowed the small, rapid pulse of cachexia for several hours with the first dose of *Digitalis purpurea*. But this is the primary action of the drug, and soon the heart beats twice as fast as before. Repeated stronger doses are less and less effective and finally do not decrease the pulse rate at all. Moreover, in the *secondary action* the pulse becomes uncountable; sleep, appetite, and strength wane, and death is imminent, or else insanity.

In a word, how often the secondary action of opposite (antipathic) remedies aggravates the disease or even produces something worse. False doctrine does not perceive this, but experience terrifyingly proves it to us.

a. M. S. Hufeland, in his paper *Homöopathie*, p. 20.

60

These unfortunate results are the natural consequence of using medicines antipathically. The orthodox physician imagines that he can get out of the difficulty by prescribing a stronger dose of the medicine with each new aggravation. This produces only another brief hushing up of the symptoms and, from the necessity to keep increasing the dose of the palliative, either some other, even worse complaint or quite often a condition of complete incurability, danger to life, even death.[a] It *never* produces a *cure* in any disease that is at all old or chronic.

a. As we see here, all the usual palliatives have a secondary action that increases the patient's suffering, and the old school physicians have to keep repeating them in stronger doses to obtain the same relief. The relief is never lasting, and the symptoms always return worse than before.

Twenty-five years ago Broussais combated, and in France ended, that senseless practice of mixing several drugs in the same prescription (for which mankind is rightly indebted to him) and, without considering homoeopathy, already widespread at the time, introduced his so-called physiological system, which *effectively* relieved the sufferings of the patient and, unlike the usual palliatives of the time, *permanently prevented all of them from returning worse than before*. And it was applicable to *all* human diseases.

Unable to bring about *true cures* and to restore health with mild, harmless medicines, Broussais found the *easier way* and more and more successfully put human sufferings to rest, time after time, *finally extinguishing the patient's life,* a treatment that unfortunately satisfied his shortsighted contemporaries.

The stronger the patient, the more conspicuous his complaints and the more lively his pain. He would whine, moan, shout, cry for help more and more loudly, until those around him could not reach the doctor quickly enough to bring him rest. All that Broussais held necessary was to weaken his patients and progressively exhaust them. The more he bled the patient and sucked out his vital fluids with his leeches and cupping glasses (for he deemed this innocent and irreplaceable blood to be the cause of nearly every suffering!), the more the patient lost his ability to feel pain and voice the aggravation of his condition with lusty complaints and gestures.

The weaker he became, the calmer he looked. The onlookers were pleased at his apparent improvement; and if the spasms, suffocation, anguish, or pain started to return, they hastened to repeat the means that had so effectively calmed him before and offered the prospects of calming him still further.

If the patient had a long-lasting disease and if he still had some strength, he was deprived of food to reduce his vitality and check his distressing condition. Very much exhausted, he was unable to protest or to prohibit further weakening of his condition through bleedings, leeches, blistering plaster, warm baths, etc. Less and less conscious of his condition, he did not realize that such *frequently repeated* reduction and draining of his life-force must end in death. And the relatives were so hypnotized by the slight relief the bleedings and tepid baths had brought to his last sufferings that they were quite surprised at the unexpected way in which he escaped from their hands. "After all, God knows, he was not treated violently on his sickbed; the slight prick of the lancet at each bleeding was hardly painful; gum arabic solution"—almost the only medicine that Broussais allowed—"was mild in taste and without visible effect; leeches bite only gently and let the prescribed amount of blood quite unnoticeably; and the tepid baths could only have been soothing. The disease must have been fatal from the very start, and the patient had to shed his mortal coil in spite of all the physician's ministrations.'' Thus the relatives of the dearly departed consoled themselves—especially those who inherited from him!

The doctors of Europe and elsewhere willingly took to this *one easy method of treating all diseases,* because it spared them all reflection (the hardest work under the sun!); and to still their pangs of conscience and console themselves to some extent, they had only to reflect that they were not, after all, the founders of this system and therapy, that thousands of other Broussais disciples did the same thing, that perhaps, as their Master had publicly taught them, everything came to an end in death, anyway. Thus thousands of doctors, forgetting the commandment of our first lawgiver—"Thou shalt shed no blood, because life is in the blood''— were wretchedly misled, and coldheartedly shed in torrents the warm blood of patients *who might have been cured.* Faithful to Broussais, they killed *gradually* more millions than Napoleon ever slew violently in battle.

Was it not perhaps ordained by Providence that this system of Broussais, *which medically killed patients who might have been cured,* should go out into the world before homoeopathy to open people's eyes to this only true art of healing, the most difficult of all arts, which, if practiced purely and conscientiously by a tireless and intelligent physician, heals all patients who are curable and gives them new life?

61

If physicians had been capable of reflecting on the sad results of applying contrary remedies, they would long since have discovered the great truth that the real and lasting art of healing must reside in the exact opposite of this antipathic way of treating disease symptoms.

They would have realized that if such medicinal action in opposition to the disease symptoms (medicine used antipathically) brings only short-lasting relief, always followed by aggravation, then the reverse, *the homoeopathic use of remedies* based on symptom similarity, must necessarily bring about a lasting, perfect cure, provided that the smallest possible doses and not large ones are given.

Neither these poor results, nor the fact that physicians obtained a lasting cure of an old or chronic disease only when perchance one of the important medicines in their prescriptions happened to act homoeopathically, nor the fact that all rapid and perfect cures ever brought about in nature (par. 46) were produced by a *similar* disease supervening upon the old one ever taught them through so many centuries this one and only right way of curing the sick.

62

The following discoveries derived from numerous observations explain the pernicious results of the palliative antipathic method and the salutary effects of the opposite, the homoeopathic method. Before me no one ever noticed them, although they were so near, so manifest, and although they were of infinite importance to the art of healing.

63

Every power that acts on life, every medicine, alters the vital force more or less and brings about in human health certain modifications of greater or lesser duration. We call this the *primary action.* Although it is a product of both the medicinal and the vital force, this primary action nevertheless belongs more to the domain of the former.

Our vital force strives to oppose its energy to this influence. This, its life-preserving reaction, is an automatic activity called *secondary action* or *counteraction.*

64

During the primary action of the artificial disease agents (medicines) on our healthy bodies, as the following examples indicate, our vital force seems to behave in a purely receptive or passive way. It is as if it were forced to receive into itself the artificial power acting from without, so allowing its state of health to be changed.

But then it seems to rally in response to this influence (*primary action*) that it has taken on.

a. It produces the exactly opposite condition (*counteraction, secondary action*) *if such a condition exists in nature.* The intensity of this reaction is proportionate to the effect (*primary action*) exerted on it by the artificial disease agent and, of course, to its own energy as well.

b. Or if such a condition directly opposite to the primary action does not exist in nature, it tries to reassert its authority by extinguishing the alteration brought about in it from without (by the medicine) and re-establishing its normal function (*secondary action, curative action*).

65

Examples of *a* abound. A hand immersed in hot water is of course at first much warmer than the other one, which is not immersed (primary action), but once removed from the hot water and completely dried it soon becomes cold, then much colder than the other hand (secondary action).

Someone who is heated by vigorous exercise (primary action) is afterward affected with cold and shivering (secondary action).

The man who yesterday was warmed by too much wine (primary action) today feels chilly from every little draft (counteraction of the organism, secondary action).

An arm that has been long immersed in the coldest water is of course at the beginning much paler and colder than the other (primary action), but removed from the cold water and dried it becomes afterward not only warmer than the other arm but even hot, red, and inflamed (secondary action, counteraction of the vital force).

Excessive liveliness results from taking strong coffee (primary action), but afterward lethargy and drowsiness remain for a long time (counteraction, secondary action) unless removed by the repeated taking of more coffee (brief palliations).

The heavy, stuporous sleep of opium (primary action) is followed on the next night by greater insomnia (counteraction, secondary action).

The constipation of opium (primary action) is followed by diarrhea (secondary action), and purging with medicines that stimulate the intestines (primary action) is followed by constipation lasting many days (secondary action).

Thus, to the primary action of every substance that in large doses strongly alters the condition of a healthy body our vital force always produces in the secondary action the exactly opposite condition (when, as stated above, such a condition exists).

66

But in a healthy body one will not notice any conspicuous secondary or counteraction to the effect of very small homoeopathic doses of pathogenetic substances.

The primary action that some of these remedies produce is perceptible to a sufficiently attentive observer, but the counteraction (secondary action) of the living organism is only as much as is needed to restore the normal condition.

67

These incontrovertible truths, which nature and experience spontaneously offer, explain to us the benefits of homoeopathic cures and, conversely, prove the absurdity of antipathic and palliative treatment with contrary remedies.[a]

a. Only in the most urgent cases, where danger to life and imminent death do not allow time for a homoeopathic remedy to act—neither hours, nor often quarter hours, nor even minutes—in sudden accidents to healthy individuals, such as asphyxiation, apparent death from lightning, choking, freezing, drowning, etc., only in such cases may we and should we as a first measure at least bring back irritability and sensitivity (physical life) by using a palliative such as gentle electrical stimulation, clysters of strong coffee, smelling salts, gradual warming, etc.

After this stimulation, the action of the vital organs resumes its former healthy course, since this was not a disease needing to be removed,* but only a restriction or inhibition of the vital energy, healthy in itself.

To this also belong various antidotes to sudden poisonings: alkalies for the ingestion of mineral acids, *Hepar sulphuris* for metal poisonings, coffee and camphor (and *Ipecacuanha*) for opium poisonings, etc.

A homoeopathic remedy is not necessarily wrongly chosen just because one or more of its symptoms is the opposite of some disease symptoms of medium or small importance, provided the remaining stronger, salient (characteristic), and peculiar symptoms of the disease are destroyed and extinguished by that same remedy through symptom similarity (homoeopathically covered and neutralized). The few opposite symptoms of the remedy disappear by themselves after it has ceased to act, without in the least delaying the cure.

68

In *homoeopathic cures* experience shows us that after the unusually small doses of medicine required in this therapy (par. 275 to par. 287), doses just sufficient to overcome the natural disease through symptom similarity and drive it from the sensation of the vital principle, it does sometimes happen that some slight medicinal disease is at first left behind *alone* in the organism. But

---

*And yet the modern mongrel sect invokes this observation (in vain) to find such exceptions to the rule everywhere and to slip in on the sly their convenient allopathic palliatives and all their other pernicious allopathic rubbish. They do this only to save themselves the trouble of looking for the correct homoeopathic remedy in each case of disease, very conveniently appearing to be homoeopathic physicians, while their *pernicious* actions prove otherwise.

because of the extraordinary minuteness of the dose, it is so fleeting and mild, and so quickly disappears by itself, that the only energy the vital force needs to exert against such a small disturbance is that required to raise the resulting state of health to one of complete cure, which, after the extinguishing of the original disease, is not much (par. 64b).

69

Exactly the opposite happens in antipathic (palliative) procedure: to counter a symptom the physician chooses an opposite medicinal symptom (e.g., opposing the primary anesthetizing action of opium to acute pain). These two symptoms are not foreign and completely allopathic to each other; there is an obvious relationship between them—an *inverse* one. The disease symptom is supposed to be destroyed by the opposite medicinal symptom, but this is impossible.

It is true that the antipathically chosen remedy touches the same diseased point in the organism as the homoeopathically chosen one. But the antipathic remedy masks the opposite natural disease symptom only superficially and hides it for a short time from the vital principle. Thus in the first moments of the palliation the vital force feels nothing disagreeable, either from the symptom or from the opposing medicinal symptom. These two forces appear mutually to have removed and, as it were, dynamically neutralized each other in the sensations of the vital principle (e.g., the anesthetizing power of opium appears to destroy the pain). The vital force feels as if it were healthy in the first minutes and is aware neither of the opiate nor of the disease pain.

But the opposite medicinal symptom *cannot* supplant the pathological untunement in the organism (in the sensations of the vital principle) as a *similar, stronger* artificial disease would do in homoeopathic procedure, cannot affect the vital principle by replacing the original natural disease with a very similar artificial one, as a homoeopathic remedy would do.

The palliative remedy produces a condition *completely different* from the pathological untunement and therefore leaves it intact. In the beginning this palliative remedy makes the vital force insensible to the natural disease, in an apparent dynamic neutralization,[a] but its effect quickly disappears by itself—all medicinal diseases do—leaving behind the natural disease unchanged.

Moreover, upon the primary action of the palliative (since all palliatives must be given in large doses to procure the appearance of relief) an opposite counteraction follows from the vital force (par. 63 to par. 65).

This secondary action, counteraction, is similar to the existing natural disease, which has not been destroyed, and must necessarily strengthen and augment it.[b]

Therefore the *disease symptom* (this individual part of the whole natural disease) *becomes worse after the action of the palliative has ceased; the larger the dose, the greater the aggravation.* To return to our example, the stronger the dose of opium given to suppress the pain, the more the pain increases over its original intensity as soon as the opium has ceased to act.[c]

a. In living people conflicting or opposite sensations are not definitively neutralized as substances of opposing properties might neutralize each other in the chemical laboratory, where, for example, sulphuric acid and potash unite to form an entirely different compound, a neutral salt, which is neither alkaline nor acidic and which, even in fire, does not break down again. As we have said, such perfect fusions producing something neutral and stable never take place and resolve opposing dynamic impressions in our sensory apparatus. There is only an appearance of neutralization and mutual annihilation for a while; the antagonistic sensations do not permanently cancel each other out. A person who is sad dries his tears for only a short time at the sight of some amusing spectacle; he soon afterward forgets this distraction, and they flow all the more copiously.

b. However clear this proposition is, it has nevertheless been misunderstood, and people have objected that "the secondary action of a palliative, being similar to the original disease, should cure just as well as the primary action of a homoeopathic medicine." They have not considered the following: the secondary action is *never* a product of the medicine, but *always* the counteraction of the vital force; therefore, from this reaction of the vital force to a palliative comes a condition similar to the disease symptom, and since the palliative has not eradicated this disease symptom, the counteraction of the vital force to the palliative then adds to it.

c. As in a dark dungeon, where the prisoner can only gradually and with difficulty distinguish his immediate surroundings, the sudden lighting of a lamp at once consolingly illuminates everything around him, but as soon as it is extinguished, the brighter the flame was, the darker the obscurity that follows, and the poor prisoner finds it far more difficult than before to see his surroundings.

70

From everything that we have said the following truths are unmistakable:

In diseases all the physician can find which is really pathological and needs to be cured consists exclusively of the patient's condition and complaints and all the changes in his health which are perceptible to the senses—in a word, of the totality of symptoms through which the disease demands the right medicine to cure it. On the other hand, every so-called inner cause of disease, every hidden condition, every imaginary material disease substance is an empty dream.

The untunement that we call disease can be changed into health only by a retuning of the vital energy through medicines whose curative virtue is nothing, therefore, but their ability to alter health, i.e., to produce symptoms in a characteristic way. And these symptoms can best and most clearly be ascertained by provings made on the healthy.

According to all experience, a natural disease can never be cured through medicines that have the inherent power to produce in the healthy a disease condition *differing* from, foreign to, the disease to be cured (dissimilar disease symptoms). Therefore allopathic therapy never cures. Even in nature it never happens that an indwelling disease is removed, destroyed, and cured by a second dissimilar one supervening upon it, no matter how strong the new one is.

Also according to all experience, medicines that have the inherent tendency to produce in the healthy an artificial disease symptom *opposite* to one that is to be cured offer only a fleeting amelioration. They never cure an older complaint—it always returns worse than before. In a word, this antipathic and purely palliative procedure brings about results exactly contrary to those desired, in serious complaints of any duration.

Finally, the only effective therapy is the third method, the only one left to consider (the *homoeopathic* one). It uses in appropriate dosage against *the totality of symptoms* of a natural disease a medicine capable of producing, in the healthy, symptoms as similar as possible. A disease is only a purely dynamic deranging stimulus; it is overcome and extinguished in the sensations of the vital principle by the similar and stronger deranging stimulus of the homoeopathic medicine—without ill effect, completely and permanently extinguished, ceasing to exist. Chance happenings in nature give us examples of this: when a new, similar disease supervenes upon an old one, the old one is quickly and permanently destroyed and healed.

71

It is clear that human diseases are nothing but groups of certain symptoms and that they are destroyed and changed into health (the process of all true cure) by means of medicinal substances, but only by those that can artificially produce similar disease symptoms.

Thus the task of curing comes down to the three following points:

I. How does the physician ascertain what he needs to know about diseases in order to cure them?

II. How does he investigate the pathogenetic power of medicines, the instruments provided for curing natural diseases?

III. How does he use these natural pathogenetic agents (medicines) most effectively to cure natural diseases?

72

The following general remarks are a preliminary consideration of the *first point* [see par. 105 and par. 146]:

Human diseases are acute or chronic.

Those we call *acute* are rapid disease processes of the abnormally untuned vital principle. They characteristically run their course and come to an end more or less quickly.

The others, insignificant and often unnoticed at the beginning, dynamically untune the living organism, each in its own way, and remove it from health gradually, in such a way that the automatic vital energy (vital force, vital principle) intended for the preservation of health can offer only imperfect, inappropriate, ineffective resistance to them, both at their start and as they continue, and can never extinguish them on its own, with its own power, so that it must impotently let them flourish while it becomes ever more untuned, until the organism is finally destroyed. We call these *chronic* diseases; they arise from the dynamic contagion of a chronic miasm.

73

There are acute diseases affecting single individuals, *diseases brought on by harmful influences* to which particular individuals have been exposed. Exciting causes of such acute febrile conditions are: excesses or privation in eating, traumatisms, chilling or overheating, fatigue, strains from lifting, etc., or else *psychic* agitation and upsets. In reality most of these acute diseases are only passing flare-ups of latent psora, which returns by itself to a dormant state if the flare-ups are not too violent and if they are quickly eliminated.

Then there are *sporadic* acute diseases, which affect a few individuals at a time here and there, acute diseases brought on by harmful meteorological or telluric influences to which only a few people are susceptible at any one time.

Bordering on these are the *epidemic* diseases, in which many individuals are affected very similarly from a similar cause. In crowded areas they tend to become *contagious*. These epidemics cause fevers, each with its own characteristics;[a] and because each case of disease in the same epidemic has the same origin, those affected manifest a similar disease process, which, left to itself, ends either in death or in recovery within a limited time. War, floods, and famine are often the exciting causes or the breeders of such diseases.

Then there are those *acute* miasms that always recur in their own particular form, which is why they are known by an established name. Some of them are contracted only once in a lifetime, like smallpox, measles, whooping cough, the old, bright red, smooth scarlatina of Sydenham,[b] mumps, etc., while others recur frequently in fairly similar ways, like the Levant plague, the yellow fever of coastal regions, Asiatic cholera, etc.

a. Physicians of the orthodox school specify only a few names for such fevers (outside of which prolific nature is not permitted to produce any others, because they want in their treatment to follow an established routine). But homoeopathic physicians are not caught in these preconceived notions of the old school and do not recognize the names jail fever, bilious fever, typhus fever, putrid fever, nerve fever, or mucous fever; they cure each according to its own characteristics, without giving it any particular name.

b. After 1801 physicians confused a certain *purpura miliaris* (*Roodvonk*), which came from the west, with scarlatina, although the characteristics of the two diseases were quite distinct. *Aconite* prevented and cured the first, which was always epidemic, *Belladonna* the second, which was most often sporadic. In the last few years these two have sometimes seemed to combine into an exanthematous fever with its own nature, for which neither of these two remedies is any longer exactly homoeopathic.

74

Among chronic diseases we must unfortunately include all those widespread illnesses artificially created by allopathic treatments, by the prolonged use of violent, heroic drugs in strong, increasing doses, the abuse of calomel, corrosive sublimate, mercurial ointment, nitrate of silver, iodine and its ointments, opium, valerian, cinchona bark and quinine, foxglove, Prussic acid, sulphur and sulphuric acid, perennial purgatives, bloodletting in torrents,[a] leeches, fontanels, setons, etc.

All these relentlessly weaken the vital force and, if they do not completely exhaust it, progressively untune it, each in its own characteristic way, to such an extent that it has to bring about a revolution in the organism to maintain life against these hostile and destructive attacks. It has to inhibit or exaggerate the excitability or sensitivity of a part of the organism, dilate or contract, soften or harden, or even completely destroy certain parts, and bring about internal or external lesions (internally and externally maiming the body) in order to protect the organism against complete destruction of life from the ever renewed hostile attacks of such ruinous forces.[b]

a. Of all therapies ever conceived, there is none more allopathic, senseless, and futile than Broussais's debilitating bloodletting and starvation diet, which have been widespread for years. No sensible man could ever find any medical benefit in such treatment, whereas a real medicinal substance, even arbitrarily chosen, has now and then helped a patient because it happened to be homoeopathic. But what can common sense expect from bloodletting other than the certain impairment and shortening of life?

To imagine that most, indeed all, diseases are only local inflammations is deplorable and completely unfounded. Even true local inflammations are most surely and quickly cured by medicines that dynamically remove the arterial irritation underlying them, without the slightest loss of vital fluids and strength, whereas bloodlettings, even directly on the affected part, only increase the tendency to renewed inflammation in these parts. Similarly, in inflammatory fevers, it is generally useless and even murderous to drain away many pounds of blood from the veins, whereas a small dose of an indicated remedy would, often in a few hours, remove the arterial irritability stirring up the blood that was previously so calm, together with the underlying disease, without the slightest loss of vital fluids and strength. Such abundant loss of blood can often not be corrected during the rest of the patient's life, because the organs intended by the Creator for the production of blood have been so deeply weakened that though they may again be able to produce the same quantity of blood, they can never produce it in the same quality.

It is impossible that this imagined plethora, which one would drain away with multiple bloodlettings, could have sprung up so suddenly, when the pulse of the patient now so feverish was so calm an hour before the paroxysm of fever. No man, no patient, ever has too much blood* or too much strength. On the

---

*The only kind of plethora to speak of occurs in a healthy woman a few days before her monthly period: she feels a certain fullness in the womb and in the breasts, without any inflammation.

contrary, every patient is lacking in strength, for if this were not so his vital principle would have warded off the disease. So it is as senseless as it is cruel (a simply murderous abuse based on a theory invented out of thin air) to inflict on an already weak patient a still greater weakness, the most severe one imaginable, by letting his blood. It does not remove his disease, which is always dynamic and can be removed only dynamically.

b. If the patient finally succumbs, at the autopsy the one who has brought such a treatment to its completion usually very cunningly presents these internal organic abnormalities brought about by his handiwork to the inconsolate relatives as the original, incurable trouble. See my book: *Allopathy: A Word of Warning to All Patients,* Leipzig, Baumgärtner [translated in *Lesser Writings*].

We find the results of such bungling illustrated in the memorably dishonest treatises of pathological anatomy. *Country folk and poor people from the cities who die of natural diseases and escape such harmful treatment are not usually subjected to autopsy.* And, to be sure, we would never find in their bodies such destruction and deformities. From this we can judge the trustworthiness of those beautiful illustrations and the integrity of these gentlemen, the book writers.

75

The ruinations of human health brought about by this pernicious allopathic treatment (at its worst in recent times) are the most tragic and most incurable of all the chronic diseases. I regret to say that when they have gone beyond a certain point it is probably impossible ever to discover or imagine any means of curing them.

76

In homoeopathy benevolent Providence has given us relief only for natural diseases.

As for the debilitation, often lasting for years, callously wrought by false practices (wasting blood and causing emaciation with setons and fontanels), and the internal and external ruinations and mutilations of the human organism from harmful and unsuitable treatments, *they would have to be removed by the life-force itself* (with appropriate help for any miasm that might be in the background), if it has not already been exhausted by these outrages and if it can devote several years to this enormous undertaking undisturbed.

No human means can ever repair those innumerable abnormalities so often produced by pernicious allopathic treatment.

77

Diseases engendered by prolonged exposure to *avoidable* noxious influences should not be called chronic. They include diseases brought about by:

the habitual indulgence in harmful food or drink;
all kinds of excesses that undermine health;
prolonged deprivation of things necessary to life;
unhealthy places, especially swampy regions;
dwelling only in cellars, damp workplaces, or other
    closed quarters;
lack of exercise or fresh air;
physical or mental overexertion;
continuing emotional stress;
etc.

These self-inflicted disturbances go away on their own with improved living conditions if no chronic miasm is present, and they cannot be called chronic diseases.

78

The true natural *chronic* diseases are those that arise from a chronic miasm and that, left to themselves without their specific remedy, continue to increase indefinitely, tormenting the patient with ever greater suffering to the end of his days, despite the best mental and dietary habits.

These diseases are by far the gravest, most numerous scourges of humanity after those caused by medical abuse (par. 74). The most robust physical constitution, the most orderly way of living, and the most lively vital energy are not equal to eradicating them.[a]

a. In the full flower of youth or at the beginning of regular menstruation, if living conditions are right for heart, mind, and body, chronic diseases often remain hidden for years. Those affected by them seem to their relatives and acquaintances to be completely healthy, and the disease acquired by contagion or inheritance seems completely to have disappeared. It is, however, inevitably brought out again in later years by adverse events or circumstances. The more the vital principle has been run down by debilitating passions, grief, and worry, and especially by unsuitable medical treatment, the more quickly it develops and the graver it is.

79

Until now only syphilis has been somewhat recognized as a chronic miasmatic disease, one that, when untreated, disappears only at death.

Sycosis (fig-wart disease), similarly ineradicable by the vital force when untreated, has not been recognized as a particular chronic miasmatic disease, which it most certainly is; it is thought to be cured with the destruction of the outgrowths on the skin, despite the lingering decline that remains.

80

Immeasurably more widespread, and consequently far more important than the two preceding, is the chronic miasm of psora.

While the other two manifest their specific chronic inner malady by the venereal chancre and the cauliflowerlike excrescences, respectively, the inner, monstrous chronic miasm of psora announces itself after the complete internal infection of the entire organism, through a characteristic cutaneous eruption accompanied by unbearably voluptuous tickling itching and a specific odor, and sometimes consisting of only a few vesicles.

This psora is the true *underlying cause* and creator of almost all the multitudinous, indeed, innumerable disease forms that are not due to syphilis and sycosis.[a]

They include: neurasthenia, hysteria, hypochondria, mania, melancholia, idiocy, madness, epilepsy and all kinds of fits, softening of the bones (rachitis), scrofula, scoliosis and kyphosis, bone caries, cancer, fungus hematodes, neoplasms, gout, hemorrhoids, jaundice and cyanosis, dropsy, amenorrhea, hemorrhage of the stomach, nose, lungs, bladder, and womb, asthma and suppuration of the lungs, impotence and infertility, migraine, deafness, cataract and amaurosis, kidney stones, paralyses, deficiencies of the senses, and every kind of pain, etc., all mentioned in pathology books as separate diseases.

a. It took me twelve years of research to find the source of this incredible number of chronic diseases, to investigate and confirm this great truth hidden from all my predecessors and contemporaries, and to discover the principal (antipsoric) remedies that are usually able to deal with this thousand-headed monster in its widely varying forms and manifestations.

My discoveries on the subject have been set forth in my book *Chronic Diseases* (4 vols., Dresden, Arnold, 1828, 1830; and 2nd ed., Düsseldorf, Schaub, in 5 vols.).

Before acquiring this knowledge I could teach my students to treat these chronic diseases only as so many different individual diseases and to use those remedies whose effects on the healthy had until then been proved. Thus in each case of chronic disease my disciples treated the group of symptoms appearing at the time as a disease in itself. They often relieved it to such a degree that sick humanity could rightly rejoice over the wealth of remedies already available to the new therapy.

But how much more reason do they have to rejoice now that they are so much nearer to the desired goal, now that I have published, with special instructions on their preparation and use, homoeopathic remedies, discovered subsequently, which are far more specific for the chronic complaints stemming from psora. The true physician can now choose from among these remedies the ones whose medicinal symptoms most homoeopathically match the chronic disease to be cured and which thus almost without exception bring about perfect cures.

81

The gradual transmission and incredible development of this ancient contagion, for hundreds of generations and through many millions of human organisms, explains to some extent the countless disease forms into which it has evolved throughout the entire human race, especially when we consider the great number of extrinsic factors[a] and the indescribable diversity of distinct congenital human constitutions that have contributed to the formation of this great variety of chronic diseases (secondary symptoms of psora).

It is no wonder that so many different, often prolonged internal and external noxious influences should produce such an endless variety of deficiencies, deteriorations, untunements, and suffering in such widely varying organisms permeated by the psoric miasm. Hitherto, the old pathology has mistakenly presented them as diseases in themselves under a multitude of particular names.[b]

a. Some of these extrinsic factors that modify the development of psora into chronic troubles are, obviously, the climate; the particular natural conditions of the place of habitation; irregularities in the physical and moral education of youth—neglect, distortion, or overrefinement; physical and moral abuses in professional or private life; diet; human passions; various morals, customs, and habits.

b. Many of these incorrect names can mean different things. The same name can describe completely different disease conditions, which often have in common only one symptom, e.g., *ague, jaundice, dropsy, consumption, leucorrhea, hemorrhoids, rheumatism, apoplexy, convulsions, hysteria, hypochondria, melancholia, mania, angina pectoris, palsy,* etc., each of which is taken to be an unchanging, fixed disease and treated according to established routine on the basis of its name.

How can a standardization of names justify a standardization of treatment; and if identical treatment is not always called for, then why use an identical name, which misleadingly implies it? *Nihil sane in artem medicam pestiferum magis unquam irrepsit malum, quam generalia quaedam nomina morbis imponere iisque aptare velle generalem quandam medicinam* ["Indeed, no more deadly evil has ever stolen into the art of medicine than the imposition of certain general names on diseases as well as the wish to adapt a certain general medicine to them."], says Huxham, whose insight and sensitive conscience command respect (*Op. phys. med.*, tome I).

Fritze (*Annalen*, vol. I, p. 80) also complains that "essentially different diseases are called by the same name."

The old school gives specific names even to those widespread acute diseases that may indeed be propagated by a specific, unknown infectious agent *within each individual epidemic*, as if they were known, fixed diseases always recurring in exactly the same form: typhus, hospital fever, jail fever, camp fever, putrid fever, typhoid fever, nerve fever, mucous fever, etc.

Yet each epidemic of such migrant fevers manifests each time as a new disease that has never before existed in exactly that form: it differs greatly in its course, in many of its most prominent symptoms, in its whole behavior. Each appearance is so dissimilar to all previous epidemics, whatever we call them, that one would have to forswear all logic and precision of thought to give such widely varying epidemics the name established by accepted pathology and to treat them all identically in accordance with this same faulty label. Only the honest Sydenham perceived this, for he insists (*Oper.*, chap. 2, *De Morb. Epid.*, p. 43) that no epidemic disease should be taken for any previous one and treated in the same way, since all that break out at different times are different from each other: *Animum admiratione percellit, quam discolor et sui plane dissimilis morborum epidemicorum facies; quae tam aperta horum morborum diversitas tum propriis ac sibi peculiaribus symptomatis tum etiam medendi ratione, quam hi ab illis disparem sibi vindicant, satis illucescit. Ex quibus constat, morbos epidemicos, utut externa quatantenus specie et symptomatis aliquot utrisque pariter convenire paullo incautioribus videantur, re tamen ipsa, si bene adverteris animum, alienae esse admodum indolis et distare ut aera lupinis.* ["It strikes the mind with wonder how different and clearly unlike one another is the appearance of epidemic diseases; there is so obvious a difference among these diseases not only in the symptoms proper and peculiar to themselves but also in the method of treating them and in the way each demands for itself a different method from any other. As a result, in whatever way and to whatever extent in external appearance and in the number of symptoms, epidemic diseases seem to agree, to those who do not pay attention; nevertheless, by the very fact itself, if one pays careful attention, these epidemic diseases are of totally different nature and are as different from one another as counterfeit money is from real money."]

From all this it is clear that a true physician will not allow these useless and incorrect disease names to influence his therapy. He knows not to judge and treat disease according to the nominal similarity of an individual symptom, but rather according to the totality of the patient's symptoms. He must carefully uncover the patient's sufferings and never jump to conclusions about them on empty hypothesis.

Nevertheless, if one still believes that now and then

it is necessary to use particular disease names in order to communicate to common people quickly when speaking about a patient, one should use them only as collective names. One might say, for example, that a patient has a *kind* of St. Vitus's dance; a *kind* of dropsy; a *kind* of nerve fever; a *kind* of ague.

One would *never* say, however (to end once and for all the confusion of these names), "*He has* St. Vitus's dance," "*He has* nerve fever," "*He has* dropsy," "*He has* ague," since there simply are not any fixed, unchanging diseases to be known by such names.

82

Although the discovery of that great source of chronic diseases, psora, and its more specific homoeopathic remedies has brought those involved in the art of healing a few steps nearer to understanding the true nature of most diseases, the homoeopathic physician must still piece together the perceptible symptoms and peculiarities of the chronic (psoric) disease being treated just as carefully as before to form an indicative picture, because no true cure of a psoric or any other kind of disease can take place without the strict individualization of every case.

In this investigation one must distinguish between acute diseases of sudden onset and chronic diseases. In the former the principal symptoms become prominent and recognizable to the senses more quickly, so the taking of the case requires far less time and there are far fewer questions to ask,[a] because most of the symptoms are self-evident; whereas in a chronic disease that has been evolving gradually for a number of years, it is far more troublesome to obtain the symptoms.

a. Therefore the following outline for searching out symptoms is only partly applicable to acute diseases.

83

This individualizing *examination of a case of disease,* which here receives only a general introduction and of which the physician will retain only what is applicable in each case, demands of the physician only impartiality, sound senses, attentive observation, and faithfulness in recording the disease picture.

84

The patient tells the history of his complaints.

The relatives describe his complaints, his behavior, and everything they have noticed about him.

The physician sees, hears, and observes with his other senses what is altered and peculiar in the patient.

He writes everything down exactly, including the verbatim expressions of patient and relatives.

Whenever possible he remains silent to let them finish what they have to say without interrupting them, as long as they do not digress unduly.[a]

At the beginning he asks them only to speak slowly so that he may write down all the essential information.

a. Every interruption disturbs the speakers' train of thought, and afterward they cannot remember exactly what they wanted to say.

85

The things the patient or his relatives say should be written down on separate lines so that all the symptoms appear separately, one above the other.

In this way the physician can add to any one of them that is too vague, in the beginning, information subsequently stated more clearly.

86

When the speakers have finished what they wanted to say, the physician adds to each individual symptom more precise information by questioning in the manner that follows. He reads through the list of symptoms and asks for particulars about this and that, e.g.:

> When did this symptom appear? Did it appear before starting this last medicine? Did it appear while taking medicine? Or not until a few days after stopping it?
>
> What was the pain in that place like? Describe exactly how it felt. Where was it exactly? Did the pain occur intermittently, at different times? Or was it persistent and continuous? How long? At what time of the day or of the night, and in what position of the body was it aggravated or else completely absent?
>
> Describe clearly the exact nature of that symptom or circumstance reported.

87

Thus the physician elicits further particulars about each of the patient's statements without ever putting words into his mouth[a] or asking a question that can be answered only by yes or no, which induces the patient to affirm something untrue or half true or else deny something really there to avoid discomfort or out of desire to please, thereby giving a wrong picture of the disease, which would lead to the wrong treatment.

a. E.g., the physician must not ask, ''Wasn't this or that circumstance also present?'' He must never be guilty in this way of suggestions leading to a false answer and a false account of the patient's condition.

88

If in the information thus far volunteered nothing has been said about several parts or functions of the body or about the disposition, the physician asks whether there is anything to be said concerning these bodily parts and functions or about the mental and affective condition of the patient.*ᵃ* But this must be done in general terms so that the person speaking is obliged to furnish details.

a. E.g.: What about going to stool? What about urination? What about sleep, during the daytime, at night? What about his feelings, his frame of mind, his memory? What is the appetite like, and the thirst? What taste is there in his mouth? Which food and drink does he most enjoy? Which does he most dislike? Do all things have their full, natural taste, or do they taste strange? How does he feel after eating or drinking? Is there anything to be said about the head, limbs, abdomen?

89

Only when the patient, whose own account of his sensations is most to be trusted (unless he is feigning illness), has finished freely relating the relevant information upon simply being invited to do so, and when the disease picture is fairly complete, may the physician ask more precise, more specific questions, as indeed he should if he feels that he has not yet been fully informed.*ᵃ a*. E.g.: How frequent are the stools? What is their exact nature? Was the white evacuation mucus or feces? Were there any pains with the evacuation? What kinds, and where exactly? What did the patient vomit up? Is the bad taste in the mouth putrid, bitter, sour, or something else? Does it come before, after, or during eating and drinking? At what time of day is it worst? What is the taste of the eructations? Is the urine cloudy on standing, or immediately after it has been passed? What color is it immediately after it has been passed? What color is the sediment?

What does the patient do during sleep, and what sounds does he make? Does he whine, moan, talk, or cry out in his sleep? Does he start in his sleep? Does he snore breathing in or breathing out? Does he lie only on his back or on his side; which side? Does he cover himself up warmly, or does he not tolerate the bedclothes? Does he wake up easily or sleep too heavily? How does he feel immediately after waking? How often does this or that complaint occur, and what brings it on each time? Does it occur while sitting, lying, standing, moving? Only on an empty stomach, or at least in the morning, or only in the evening, or only after eating—or when?

When does the chill occur? Is it only a sensation of coldness, or is he also objectively cold? In what parts? Or is he actually hot to the touch while he feels a sensation of coldness? Is it only a sensation of coldness without shivering? Is he hot without having a flushed face? In what parts is he hot to the touch? Does he complain of heat without being hot to the touch? How long does the chill last? How long does the heat last?

When does he become thirsty? During the chill? During the heat? Or before or after? How thirsty is he? What is he thirsty for?

When does he sweat? At the beginning or at the end of the heat? Or how many hours after? During sleep or waking? How much does he sweat? Hot or cold? On what parts of the body? How does it smell?

What does he complain of before or during the chill; during the heat; after it; during or after the sweat?

In women, what are the monthly flow and other discharges like?

90

When the physician has written down these statements, he records what he himself observes in the patient[a] and determines how much of this was present before the illness.

a. E.g.: How has the patient been behaving during the consultation? Has he been unpleasant, quarrelsome, hurried, tearful, anxious, despondent or sad, cheerful, calm, etc.? Is he drowsy or completely unconscious? Is his voice hoarse, quiet? Has he been speaking incoherently or in some other way? What color are his face, his eyes, his skin in general? Does he have life and strength in his expression, in his eyes? What about the tongue, the respiration, the odor of the breath, the hearing? To what extent are the pupils dilated or contracted? How quickly and to what extent do they respond to different levels of illumination? What is the pulse like? What is the abdomen like? How moist or dry, how cold or hot to the touch is the skin in particular parts or in general? Does he lie with his head thrown back; with his mouth half or completely open; with his arms above his head; on his back; in some other position? How difficult is it for him to sit up? Is there anything else that strikes the physician?

91

The symptoms and feelings of a patient just after a previous course of medicine do not give the true picture of the disease.

On the other hand the symptoms and complaints from which he suffered *before taking the medicines or several days after having discontinued them* are the ones that give the true, fundamental idea of the *original* form of the disease. These are the ones the physician must especially record.

If the disease is chronic and if the patient has been taking medicine until then, the physician could also leave him entirely without medicine for a few days or give him something nonmedicinal for the time being, postponing until later the more detailed examination of the case so that he will be able to see the lasting, unmixed symptoms of the old complaint in their purity and record a faithful picture of the disease.

92

If, on the other hand, the disease is a rapidly developing one and so urgent that it will not permit any delay, the physician must be content to consider it as it is, even altered by medicines, if he cannot discover what the symptoms were before. He can then put together a complete picture of the disease, at least in its present form (the medicinal disease combined with the original one), which has usually been made graver and more dangerous than the original one by wrong treatment and which for that reason often urgently needs effective treatment. And he will then be able to overcome the disease with the appropriate homoeopathic remedy and save the patient from dying from the harmful medicine he has taken.

93

If the disease has been brought on by some noteworthy event, recently or, in the case of a chronic affection, some time ago, the patient will report it either spontaneously or upon careful questioning; or, failing that, the relatives will report it when questioned privately.[a]

a. Anything shameful that has precipitated the disease and that the patient or the relatives do not volunteer or willingly divulge the physician should try to uncover by adroitly phrased questions or by other inquiries made in private. Among such things are the following: attempted suicide or poisoning; onanism; intemperate indulgence in the passions or unnatural passions; overindulgence in wine, liqueurs, and other alcoholic drinks, tea or coffee; overindulgence in eating generally and in especially harmful foods; venereal disease or scabies; unhappiness in love; jealousy; domestic strife; vexation; tragedy in the family; grief over being subjected to abuse; suppressed resentment; wounded pride; loss of fortune; superstitious fears; hunger; some defect in the private parts—hernia, prolapse; etc.

94

While taking a case of chronic disease one should carefully examine and weigh the particular conditions of the patient's day-to-day activities, living habits, diet, domestic situation, and so on. One should ascertain whether there is anything in them which may cause or sustain the disease and remove it to help the cure.[a]

a. In chronic diseases in women one should pay particular attention to such things as pregnancy, infertility, sexual desire, confinement, miscarriages, nursing, vaginal discharges, and the condition of the monthly flow, especially noting whether it recurs at intervals that are too short or too long, how many days it lasts, whether or not it is interrupted, the quantity, how dark the color, any leucorrhea before or after the flow, and, above all, any complaints of body or psyche, any sensations or pains before, during, or after the flow. If there is leucorrhea, what is it like, what sensations accompany it, what is its quantity, under what conditions does it appear, what brings it on?

95

In chronic diseases the investigation of the symptoms mentioned above, and of all others, should be conducted as carefully and thoroughly as possible, and one should pay attention to the smallest details, partly because they are most characteristic and significant in chronic diseases and most different from those of acute diseases and cannot be too carefully considered if one is to achieve a cure, and partly because patients become so accustomed to prolonged suffering that they no longer pay much, if any, attention to the many smaller concomitant circumstances, which are often very significant (characteristic) and decisive in the search for the remedy, considering them almost to be a part of their natural condition, almost health itself, for after fifteen or twenty years of suffering they have nearly forgotten how health really feels. It hardly occurs to them that these less troublesome symptoms, which are greater or lesser deviations from health could have anything to do with their chief complaint.

96

Patients themselves are of widely varying temperaments: some, especially the so-called hypochondriacs and also others who are very sensitive and intolerant of pain, present their complaints too vividly and use exaggerated expressions to encourage the physician to help them.[a]

a. Not even the most extreme hypochondriacs will entirely fabricate their complaints and symptoms: we see this when we compare the complaints they present at different times while the physician prescribes nothing or prescribes something entirely nonmedicinal. One makes allowances for their exaggeration or at least attributes the intensity of their delivery to an excess of feeling; the high-pitched description of their suffering should itself be considered important among the symptoms that together make up the disease picture.

Insane and malicious patients who fabricate their diseases are a very different matter.

97

There are others of the opposite nature, who keep back a number of complaints— either from indolence, from misplaced modesty, from a certain mildness of disposition, or from backwardness—and describe them with vagueness or present some of them as being unimportant.

98

Since the physician must pay particular attention to what the patient himself says about his complaints and sensations, and especially the exact expressions the patient uses to describe them—because in the mouths of relatives and attendants they often become altered and distorted—uncovering the true, complete, detailed picture of any disease, but especially of a chronic one, requires a high degree of tact, consideration, knowledge of human nature, care in questioning, and patience.

99

On the whole it will be easier for the physician to take the case in diseases that are acute or that have arisen recently, because all the symptoms and deviations from the healthy condition, which was only recently lost, are to patient and relatives still fresh in the memory, still new and striking.

The physician must of course know everything here also, but he needs to *probe* far less, because everything he needs to know is told to him, most of it spontaneously.

100

In investigating the totality of symptoms of epidemics and sporadic diseases, it makes no difference at all whether something similar, by the same or a different name, has ever appeared in the world before.

Whether or not such an epidemic is new or unusual makes no difference either in the examination or in the cure, since in any case the physician must presume the true picture of every epidemic to be new and unknown and must thoroughly examine it as it is in all its details if he wants to be a true and thorough physician who never replaces observation with guesswork, who never lets himself assume that the treatment of any given case in his care is wholly or partly known in advance and that he need not carefully seek out all its expressions.

This is all the more necessary because every epidemic is in many ways unique and upon careful examination is found to be very different from all previous ones falsely bearing the same name, the only exceptions being those caused by the same unvarying infectious agent, such as smallpox, measles, etc.

101

Usually the physician does not immediately perceive the complete picture of the epidemic in the first case that he treats, since each collective disease reveals itself in the totality of its signs and symptoms only after several cases have been closely observed. Nevertheless, an observant physician can often come so close after seeing only one or two patients that he becomes aware of the characteristic picture of the epidemic and can already find its appropriate homoeopathic remedy.

102

From writing down the symptoms of several cases of this sort, the outline of the disease picture becomes more and more complete—not more extensive and wordy, but more characteristic, containing more accurately the peculiarity of the particular collective disease. The ordinary symptoms—e.g., loss of appetite, sleeplessness, etc.—become more precisely qualified, and those that are more exceptional, special, and, in the circumstances, unusual, and belong to only a few diseases, reveal themselves and constitute the characteristic picture of this epidemic.[a]

All those who catch an epidemic at a particular time have a disease flowing from the same source and therefore the *same* disease. But the entire scope of such an epidemic disease, the totality of its symptoms (which we need to know in order to grasp the whole disease picture and choose an appropriate homoeopathic remedy for it) cannot be perceived in any one patient, but can be fully distilled and gathered only from the sufferings of several patients with different physical constitutions.

a. In subsequent cases either the appropriateness of the homoeopathic remedy chosen in the first cases will be corroborated or else a more appropriate one, *the most appropriate one,* will be revealed to the physician.

103

This same method that I have taught for epidemic diseases—usually acute—I have had to apply much more precisely than ever before to essentially unvarying miasmatic chronic diseases as well, principally psora.

These chronic diseases must be investigated in the entire range of their symptoms. Any one patient takes on only a part of a chronic disease, while a second and a third, etc., suffer from some of its other symptoms, other parts as it were plucked from the totality of symptoms that make up the whole extent of the same chronic disease.

Thus the totality of symptoms of such a miasmatic chronic disease, especially psora, can be established only from *very many individual cases.*

Without such an overview and total picture, the medicines that will homoeopathically heal the entire chronic illness (e.g., the antipsorics) and are at the same time the true remedies for individual patients suffering from it cannot be sought out.

104

When the picture of any case of disease, i.e., the totality of symptoms particularly defining and distinguishing it, is precisely written down,[a] then the most difficult part of the task is already accomplished.

In his treatment, especially of chronic disease, the physician can always refer to it. He can peruse it in all its parts and pick out the characteristic symptoms so as to counter them, i.e., counter the complaint itself, with the appropriately similar artificial disease agent, the homoeopathic remedy chosen from the symptom lists of all the medicines whose pure effects have been ascertained.

And when during the treatment he inquires about the effect of the medicine and the changes in the patient's health and records his findings in his casebook, all he needs to do is omit from the original set of symptoms written down at the beginning those that are cured, note those that are still present, and add any new ones that may have arisen.

a. The physician of the old school made it extremely comfortable for himself in this regard. He did not make precise inquiries into all the circumstances of the case; indeed, he often even interrupted the patient who was describing his individual complaints, so that he would not be distracted in quickly writing the prescription, which was composed of several ingredients whose true effects were unknown to him.

As we have said, no allopathic physician ever

wanted to know all the precise circumstances of a case, and *much less did he ever write any of them down*. When he saw the patient again several days later he knew little or nothing of the few particulars he had heard before (since he had seen so many different patients in the meantime); what he had heard had gone in one ear and out the other. During subsequent visits, also, he asked only a few general questions, made as if to take the pulse at the wrist, looked at the tongue, and wrote in the same few seconds, as senselessly as before, another prescription or had the first one continued (usually in substantial doses several times a day), and then prettily hurried off to the fiftieth or sixtieth patient whom he had to visit with equal frivolity in the same morning.

And this is how people who called themselves doctors, *rational physicians,* practiced what is really the gravest of all occupations, the conscientious and careful investigation of every individual case and the appropriate therapy based on it. Naturally their results were bad, almost without exception. But patients had to go to them, partly because there was nothing better, partly out of fashion and established convention.

105

The *second point* [see par. 72 and par. 146] is that the true physician must *investigate the tools intended for the cure of natural diseases,* he must investigate the pathogenetic power of medicines so that in order to heal he may choose one having in its set of symptoms ones that constitute an artificial disease as similar as possible to the main symptom complex of the natural disease being treated.

106

One must know the entire pathogenetic action of individual remedies.

In other words, all the pathological symptoms and changes in health which each specifically can bring about in the healthy must first be observed before one can hope to find and choose from among them the correct homoeopathic remedies for most natural diseases.

107

If one tries to make this investigation by giving medicines only to *sick* people, even if each medicine is administered unmixed and alone, one sees little or nothing conclusive of their pure effects, because the specific alterations in health which they can be expected to bring about can only rarely be clearly perceived when they are mixed up with the symptoms of the natural disease already present.

108

There is no other possible way of correctly ascertaining the characteristic action of medicines on human health—no single surer, more natural way—than administering individual medicines experimentally to *healthy* people in moderate doses in order to ascertain what changes, symptoms, and effects each in particular brings about in the body and the psyche, i.e., which disease elements it can produce and tends to produce.[a]

As pointed out before (par. 24 to par. 27), all the healing virtues of medicines lie exclusively in this, their power to change human health, and this power to cure is revealed by the observation of these effects.

a. In the last three thousand five hundred years, not one single physician, to my knowledge, no one but the great, immortal *Albrecht von Haller,* has come upon this so natural, so absolutely necessary, so uniquely valid proving of the pure, characteristic action of medicines—their ability to alter human health—in order to ascertain which disease conditions each of them is capable of curing.

Although not a practicing physician, he was the only one before me who perceived the necessity of this. (See the foreword to his *Pharmacopoeia Helvet.,* Basel, 1771, fol., p. 12: *Nempe primum in corpore* sano *medela tentanda est,* sine peregrina ulla miscela; *odoreque et sapore ejus exploratis, exigua illius dosis ingerenda et ad omnes, quae inde contingunt, affectiones, quis pulsus, qui calor, quae respiratio, quaenam excretiones, attendendum. Inde ad ductum phaenomenorum, in sano obviorum, transeas ad experimenta in corpore aegroto,* etc.) ["Indeed, a remedy must first of all be essayed in a *healthy* body, *without any foreign admixture;* when the odor and taste of the remedy have been examined, a small dose of it must be taken, and attention must be paid to each change that occurs thereafter, what the pulse is, what the temperature is, the respiration, and the excretions. Then, after the examination of symptoms encountered in the healthy person, one may proceed to the trials in the body of an ill person."]

But *no one, not a single physician,* paid attention to his invaluable hint or followed it.

109

I was the first to tread this path. And my steadfastness of purpose came about and was sustained only because I was completely convinced of the great truth and blessing to mankind that the homoeopathic use of medicines was the only certain way in which it was possible to cure human diseases.[a,b]

a. I published the first fruits of this labor, as ripe as they could be at that time, in the *Fragmenta de viribus medicamentorum positivis, sive in sano corpore humano observatis* [Fragments concerning the positive force of medicines, or, more accurately, the force of medicines observed in the healthy human body], Lipsiae, 1805, pts. I, II, vol. 8, ap. J. A. Barth; the riper fruits in *Reine Arzneimittellehre,* vol. I, 3rd ed.; vol. II, 3rd ed., 1833; vol. III, 2nd ed., 1825; vol. IV, 2nd ed., 1825; vol. V, 2nd ed., 1826; vol. VI, 2nd ed., 1827 [English translation, *Materia Medica Pura,* vols. I and II]; and in the second, third, and fourth parts of *Die chronischen Krankheiten,* 1828, 1830, Dresden, Arnold (2nd ed., with a fifth part, Düsseldorf, Schaub, 1835 to 1839) [English translation, *Chronic Diseases*].

b. There could not possibly be any true, best way of curing dynamic (i.e., all nonsurgical) diseases other than pure homoeopathy, just as one could not possibly draw more than one straight line between two given points.

How superficially one must understand homoeopathy if one imagines that there are any other methods of curing diseases, how carelessly one must practice it, how few proper homoeopathic cures one must have seen or read about; and conversely, how little one must have reflected on the baselessness of every allopathic treatment of disease or inquired into its bad and equally often horrible results to put the only true art of healing on a par with these harmful treatments with such lax indifference or even to present them as indispensable adjuvants to homoeopathy! My conscientious disciples, the genuine, pure homoeopaths, with their almost always perfect, successful cures, might teach such people better.

110

Moreover, I found from the toxicological reports of earlier writers that the effects of large quantities of noxious substances ingested by healthy people—either inadvertently, or from intent to kill self or others, or for other reasons—largely coincided with my own findings from experiments with those substances on myself and on other healthy people. These writers recorded these previous cases as toxicological reports and as demonstrations of the harmfulness of these virulent substances, usually only as warnings, also to boast of the skill with which they brought about gradual recovery from these dangerous incidents with their own treatment, and also, when people thus afflicted died during treatment, to exonerate themselves by proclaiming the dangerousness of these substances, which they then called poisons.

None of these observers had any idea that the symptoms they described, exclusively to show the harmfulness and toxicity of these substances, held the positive indication of the power of these drugs to extinguish the similar complaints of natural diseases therapeutically; none suspected that these pathological disturbances were the indication of their curative homoeopathic action or that the observation of such changes that the medicines brought about in the condition of healthy bodies constituted the only possible way of finding their medicinal virtues.

The pure, characteristic, curative virtues of medicines cannot be apprehended by specious a priori sophistry, or from the smell, taste, or appearance of the medicines, or from chemical analysis, or by treating disease with one or more of them in a mixture (prescription).

Nobody had any idea that these reports of medicinal diseases would some day turn out to be the rudimentary beginnings of the true, pure materia medica. From the earliest beginnings until now, the materia medica has consisted only of false suppositions and fancies, which is as good as no materia medica at all.[a]

a. See what I have said on this subject in the "Examination of the Sources of the Ordinary Materia Medica," prefixed to the third volume of my *Reine Arzneimittellehre* [translated in *Materia Medica Pura*, vol. II].

111

The agreement of my own observations of pure medicinal effects with these earlier observations—even though the latter were written down without regard to their therapeutic value—and even the agreement among different authors of such reports, easily convinces us that medicinal substances pathologically alter healthy human bodies *according to definite, eternal, natural laws* and that by virtue of these laws *each substance can produce those specific, fixed, reliable disease symptoms that are characteristic of it.*

112

In these earlier descriptions of the effects, often life threatening, of medicines taken immoderately in this way, one also comes across conditions that manifest themselves, not at the beginning of these sad events, but toward the end, and that are in nature entirely opposite to those that manifested themselves at the beginning.

These symptoms, opposite to the *primary* (par. 63) or true action of the medicines on the vital force, are the counteraction of the organism's vital principle, its *secondary action* (par. 62 to par. 67).

In moderate doses tested on healthy organisms, however, there is seldom if ever any sign of them, and in small doses never any sign at all. During homoeopathic therapy the counteraction of the living organism to these small doses is only as great as is needed to re-establish the natural healthy state.

113

Only narcotics seem to be an exception. In their primary action they take away sensation, sensitivity, or irritability, and in moderate experimental doses on the healthy it usually does happen that there is a noticeable increase in sensitivity and irritability during the *secondary action.*

114

Apart from narcotics, in experiments with moderate doses on the healthy, one notices only the primary effects of the medicine, i.e., those symptoms with which it disturbs human health and creates in it a pathological condition of greater or lesser duration.

115

In the primary action of some medicines there are several symptoms that are in part or in certain details opposite to other previous or subsequent symptoms.

But we should not for this reason consider them to be

a true *secondary action* or a simple counteraction of the vital force; rather, we should consider them to be paroxysms, alternating in nature, within the primary action. We call this an *alternating action*.

116

Some symptoms are produced by medicines frequently, i.e., in many organisms; others are produced less frequently, in a few people; some are produced only in very few healthy organisms.

117

What we call idiosyncracies belong to the last category.

We mean that particular physical disposition, in otherwise healthy persons, to become more or less sick from certain things that do not *appear* to make any impression or alteration at all on many other people.[a]

This absence of effect in some people is only apparent. In idiosyncracies, as in all other pathological changes in human health, two things are required: the inherent power of the substance acting and the ability of the spirit-like *dynamis* (vital principle) animating the organism to react to it. From this it follows that the striking illnesses that we call idiosyncracies must be attributed not only to particular physical constitutions but also to the things that bring them on. These latter must have the power to effect the same influence on all humans, except that only a few healthy physical constitutions have the propensity to be made so noticeably ill by them.

We can see that these substances really do work this

influence on everybody because they act on *all* sick people as homoeopathic remedies for disease symptoms similar to those that they can produce, even though they actually produce them visibly only in so-called idiosyncratic people.[b]

a. There are people who faint from the smell of roses and others who can become sick in many other ways, sometimes dangerously, from eating mussels, crab, barbel roe, from touching the leaves of some varieties of sumac, etc.

b. Princess Maria Porphyrogeneta helped her brother, the Emperor Alexius, who suffered from fainting fits, by spraying him with rose water in the presence of his aunt Eudoxia (τὸ τῶν ῥόδων στάλαγμα). [The Greek here literally means: "The liquid drop of the roses."] (*Hist. byz. Alexias,* lib. XV, p. 503, ed. Posser); and Horstius (*Oper.,* III, p. 59) held that rose vinegar was helpful for fainting fits.

118

Every medicine exhibits in the human body specific effects that do not occur from any other medicinal substance in exactly the same way.[a]

a. The excellent A. von Haller saw this also, since he said (preface to his *Hist. stirp. helv.*): *Latet immensa virium diversitas in iis ipsis plantis, quarum facies externas dudum novimus, animas quasi et quodcunque caelestius habent, nondum perspeximus.* ["A great diversity of strength lies hidden in these plants themselves, whose external features we have long known but whose souls, as it were, and whatever divine element they have, we have not yet perceived.''

119

Just as certainly as every kind of plant is different from every other family and species of plant in its outer form, in the particular way in which it lives and grows, in its taste and smell; just as certainly as every mineral and every salt is different from every other in its external as well as its inner physical and chemical properties (which in itself should have prevented all confusion among them), so also it is certain that these plants and minerals are all different and distinct from each other in their pathogenetic and therefore curative effects.[a]

Each of these substances acts in its own distinct, appointed way to produce modifications in human health and feelings, so that it is impossible to mistake one for another.[b]

a. Anybody who completely understands how remarkably distinct the effects of every individual substance on the human economy are from the effects of any other and realizes the importance of this easily sees that medically speaking no one of them can ever be equivalent to any other—there can be no *surrogates*.

Only one who does *not* know the pure, positive effects of the different medicines could be so foolish as to have us believe that one could be used in the place of another and do just as well in the same disease. This is the way in which ignorant children confuse essentially different things because they hardly even know them outwardly and know them far less by their worth, their true meaning, their inner, highly distinctive properties.

b. If this is the exact truth—which it is—henceforth no doctor who does not want to be taken for an idiot and who does not want to violate his conscience, the sole arbiter of true human dignity, could possibly treat a disease with any medicinal substance unless he knows its true value precisely and completely, unless he has sufficiently tested its real effects on healthy people to know beyond doubt that it can produce a disease condition very similar to the one to be cured, more similar than that of any other medicine he knows. As pointed out above, neither man nor great nature can cure perfectly, quickly, and permanently in any way except homoeopathically.

No true physician can ever again dispense with such experiments, especially on himself, if he is to acquire this knowledge of medicines so essential for healing, this knowledge so contemptuously neglected by physicians of all past centuries.

All past centuries—posterity will hardly believe this—were content to prescribe for diseases in this blind way, to prescribe medicines of unknown value, which had *never been proved* to ascertain their highly important, highly distinct, pure dynamic action on human health. Indeed, they generally prescribed several of these unknown, very different forces all mixed together. What would happen to the patient after this they left to *chance.*

It is rather as if a madman were to force his way into an artist's workshop and grab *handfuls of different tools unfamiliar to him* to work on the art around him—so he thought. One need hardly say that this mad treatment would ruin the works of art, probably beyond all repair.

120

So medicines, upon which depend people's life and death, health and disease, must be nicely, very exactly distinguished from each other and therefore proved on the healthy through careful, pure experiments in order to ascertain their virtues and true effects.

All this is necessary in order for the physician to become thoroughly acquainted with them and to avoid any errors in using them to treat diseases, because only a correctly chosen remedy can quickly and permanently restore that greatest of all earthly blessings, well-being of body and soul.

121

In proving medicines to ascertain their effects on the healthy organism, one must bear in mind that

strong, so-called heroic substances bring about alterations in health even in small doses, even on robust people;

milder ones must be given in larger doses in these experiments;

the weakest ones, on the other hand, reveal their true action only when tested on delicate, susceptible, and sensitive people who are free from disease.

122

In such experiments—on which the certainty of the entire art of healing and the well-being of all future generations of mankind depend—no medicines should be taken but those that one knows thoroughly, those whose purity, authenticity, and full potency one is completely certain of.

123

Each of these medicines must be taken in completely simple, unrefined form:

Indigenous plants: the freshly expressed juice mixed with a little wine spirit* to prevent spoiling.

Nonindigenous plants: in powder or else a tincture of the fresh plant in wine spirit, to which a few parts of water have then been added.

Salts and gums: dissolved in water immediately before use.

If the plant is available only in dry form and is by nature without much strength, for such an experiment it is enough to use an infusion made by pouring boiling water on the crushed herb. This infusion must be taken immediately after preparation, while still hot, because all expressed plant juices and all aqueous infusions of vegetable substances quickly ferment and spoil without the addition of alcohol and lose their medicinal power.

124

For this purpose each medicinal substance must be used completely on its own and in entirely pure form, without the admixture of any foreign substance. Nothing else of a foreign medicinal nature is to be taken on the same day nor on subsequent days for as long as one wishes to observe the effects of the medicine.

*[See translators' note to par. 270.]

125

During the experiment the diet must be carefully regulated. It should consist as much as possible of simple, nourishing food without spices, and one should avoid green side dishes, roots, all salads, and soup herbs (all of which always retain some disturbing medicinal properties no matter how they are prepared).[a]

Beverages should be those usually taken and should as much as possible not be stimulants.[b]

a. Young green peas in the pod, green beans, steamed potatoes, and, if need be, carrots can be eaten. They are permissible as the least medicinal vegetables.

b. The subject of the experiment must not be in the habit of taking wine, spirits, coffee, or tea and should long before have given up the use of these stimulating, medicinally harmful beverages completely.

126

The person chosen for the experiment must *above all* be *trustworthy* and *conscientious*. During the experiment he must guard against all overexertion of body and mind and all excesses and disturbing passions.

No urgent duties must keep him from making the necessary observations. He must be willing to observe himself with close attentiveness and must be allowed to remain undisturbed while doing so. He must possess what is for him physical health and also the necessary intelligence to be able to name and describe his sensations clearly.

127

Medicines must be proved on males and females in order to bring to light those changes in health in which gender is relevant.

128

The latest discoveries, as well as earlier ones, have shown that crude medicinal substances when taken by the prover to test their characteristic effects do not express the full range of their latent hidden powers nearly as much as those taken in high dilutions correctly potentized by trituration and succussion. By this simple process the virtues hidden and, as it were, lying dormant in their crude state are developed to an unbelievable degree and roused to activity.

Today the best way to investigate the medicinal virtues of substances, even those considered weak, is to have the subject take on an empty stomach, daily for several days, four to six very fine granules of the thirtieth potency of the substance moistened with a little water or, better still, dissolved in water and thoroughly shaken.

129

When only weak effects appear from such a dose one can increase it daily by a few granules until the effects become clearer and stronger and the changes in health more perceptible.

Not all people are equally strongly affected by a medicine; on the contrary, there are great variations in this regard. For instance, a person who seems weak will sometimes hardly be affected by moderate doses of a medicine known to be very strong but will be affected strongly enough by various other much weaker ones.

Conversely, there are very strong people who feel very marked disease symptoms from an apparently mild medicine and lesser ones from stronger medicines, etc.

Since one cannot know this in advance, it is highly advisable to start with a small dose of medicine for everybody and, where appropriate and necessary, increase it from day to day.

130

If one gives, right at the beginning and for the first time, a dose of medicine in the correct strength, one has the advantage that the subject of the experiment will experience the chronology of the symptoms and be able to write down the exact time at which each appears. This teaches us much about the character of the medicine, because then the sequence of the primary effects and of the alternating effects is most unambiguous.

Even a very moderate dose is often sufficient for the experiment if the subject is sensitive enough and as attentive as possible to the way he feels.

The duration of the action of a medicine becomes known only after several experiments have been compared.

131

If in the experiment one has to give the same medicine in ever-increasing doses to the same subject for a number of consecutive days in order to obtain any result, one does, to be sure, elicit the many different disease conditions that this medicine in general can produce, but not their sequence; a later dose often removes one or another of the symptoms caused by an earlier one, either curatively or by producing the opposite condition. These symptoms must be noted in parentheses as being ambiguous—until such time as subsequent, purer experiments show whether they are counteractions, secondary actions, of the organism or the alternating action of the medicine.

132

When, however, one wants to investigate only the symptoms themselves, and not their order of appearance, or the duration of the action of the medicine, then—especially with a substance of weak action—it is preferable to increase the dose daily for several days. In this way the effect of an unknown medicine, even the mildest, will be revealed, especially if tested on sensitive subjects.

133

In order to define a particular medicinal symptom with precision, it is helpful and indeed necessary when experiencing it to place oneself in varying circumstances and to observe whether it increases, decreases, or disappears from movement of the affected part, from walking indoors or in the open, from standing, sitting, or lying; whether or not it tends to return when one reverts to the earlier circumstances; whether it is modified by such things as eating, drinking, speaking, coughing, sneezing, or other bodily activities; at what time of day or night it tends to be particularly evident. In this way the individual characteristics of a symptom become apparent.

134

All external forces, and especially medicines, have the propensity to produce specific changes in the health of the living organism in their own characteristic way.

But the symptoms proper to a medicine do not all come out in one subject, or immediately, or in the same experiment: in one subject certain symptoms are prominent in the first experiment, other symptoms in the second or third experiment, while in other subjects different symptoms are prominent. Some that occur in the second, sixth, or ninth subject might reappear in the fourth, eighth, or tenth, etc., and not always at the same hour.

135

The total picture of disease symptoms that a medicine can produce approaches completion only after multiple observations have been made on many suitable persons of both sexes, with various constitutions.

One can be sure that one has exhaustively proved a medicine and revealed the disease states that it can produce, i.e., its pure powers to alter human health, only when people who prove it later notice in it little that is new—almost always symptoms already observed by others.

136

As we have said, in provings on the healthy the changes in health which a medicine can produce cannot all be brought out in any one person, but only in many different people of various physical and psychic constitutions. Nevertheless, it does have the tendency to produce all of these symptoms in everybody (par. 117), according to an eternal, immutable law of nature. This law provides that when the medicine is administered to a person who is sick with similar symptoms, it will exert all its powers, even those that it has seldom revealed in the healthy.

When homoeopathically chosen, it then silently produces in the patient, even in the minutest dose, an artificial condition approximating the natural disease and quickly and permanently cures and frees him (homoeopathically) of his trouble.

137

If one takes pains to facilitate the investigation by choosing a truthful, sensitive subject, one who is temperate in all matters and who observes himself with the most scrupulous attentiveness, the more moderate the doses of medicine used for such experiments (up to a certain point), the more clearly do the primary effects appear, and only these, the ones most worth knowing, without any secondary effects or countereffects of the vital principle. On the other hand, when the medicine is given in excessively large doses, not only do several secondary effects appear as well among the symptoms, but the primary effects come on with such confusing rapidity and such violence that nothing can be precisely observed, not to mention that it is dangerous—something that cannot be a matter of indifference to anybody who respects mankind and counts even the lowliest of men as his brother.

138

If the previously mentioned requirements for a good, pure experiment have been fulfilled (par. 124 to par. 127), all complaints, symptoms, and changes in health of the experimental subject during the action of the medicine arise only from the medicine and must be regarded and recorded as belonging characteristically to it—must be regarded as its symptoms, even if the person has noticed similar symptoms in himself *a considerable time before*. Their reappearance during the testing of the medicine indicates only that the subject is especially predisposed to them by his particular physical constitution. As far as we are concerned, this happens because of the medicine: symptoms that come on at this time, while the powerful medicine dominates the subject's economy, arise from the medicine and not spontaneously.

139

If the physician has not himself taken the medicine for purposes of experiment but has given it to someone else, then that person must write down clearly all his sensations, complaints, attacks, and changes in health the moment they occur, noting the time elapsed between the taking of the medicine and the appearance of each symptom and also, if the symptom lasts a long time, its duration.

The physician examines the record in the presence of the subject immediately after the experiment is completed or every day if it lasts for several days and questions him, while everything is still fresh in his memory, about the exact nature of each statement written down so that he may qualify or amend it from what the subject says.[a]

a. Anybody publishing the results of such experiments for the medical world becomes responsible for the reliability of the experimental subject and the accuracy of his reports, and rightly so, since the well-being of suffering mankind is at stake.

140

If the subject cannot write, the physician must find out from him every day what has happened to him and the way in which it has happened. This report should as much as possible be the subject's own spontaneous account. None of the findings recorded should be guesswork or imagination, and they should as little as possible be obtained by close questioning: everything should be subjected to the precautions already specified (par. 84 to par. 99) for taking cases and forming pictures of natural diseases.

141

But of all the provings of the pure effects of simple medicines in altering human health and of the artificial disease conditions and symptoms that they can produce in the healthy, the best will always be those that the healthy, unprejudiced, conscientious, sensitive *physician* undertakes *on himself,* with all the precautions and care that I have taught him here. He knows with the greatest certainty what he has perceived in himself.[a]

a. These self-provings have other irreplaceable advantages for the physician. Firstly, they bring home to him irrefutably the great truth that what is medicinal in all medicines, the basis of their therapeutic value, lies in the disease conditions and changes in health which he has experienced in proving them.

Secondly, such noteworthy observations on himself lead him to an understanding of his own sensations, the way he thinks and feels (the essence of all true wisdom: γνῶθι σεαυτόν) ["know thyself"]; furthermore—something no physician can dispense with—they make him an observer. None of the observations we make on others are nearly as interesting as those we make on ourselves. In observing others one must always fear the possibility that the subject of the experiment may not have felt entirely clearly what he said or that he might not have described what he felt in exactly the right words. One can never be sure that one has not been deceived, at least to some extent. These obstacles to knowing the truth, which can never be completely overcome when one investigates the artificial disease symptoms of medicines in others, disappear entirely in self-provings. The self-prover knows without any doubt what he himself has felt, and each proving is for him further incentive to investigate the power of other medicines.

By continuing to observe himself, a more reliable, undeceiving subject, he becomes more and more skilled in the art of observation, which is so important for the physician, and he will pursue it all the more enthusiastically since these experiments on himself promise reliable knowledge of the true worth and meaning of the instruments of cure, most of which are still incompletely known.

Let him not imagine that the indispositions suffered from proving medicines could be at all harmful to his health. On the contrary, experience shows that these repeated assaults on the healthy economy of the prover only make his organism better at warding off everything inimical in his environment, all artificial and natural disease agents, and also more resistant to any harmful effects of the controlled self-provings. His health becomes more invariable; he becomes more robust. All experience shows this.

142

Distinguishing symptoms produced by a simple medicine from those of the disease that it was taken to cure demands the highest discernment and must be left strictly to master observers, especially if the disease is a slow, chronic one.[a]

   a. Symptoms that were never before noticed, or that were perhaps noticed much earlier in the disease, are new ones belonging to the medicine.

143

If one has tested a considerable number of simple medicines on healthy people in this way and has carefully and faithfully recorded all the manifestations and symptoms that they can of their own accord produce as artificial disease agents, then one has for the first time a *true materia medica:* a collection of the authentic, pure, reliable[a] effects of simple medicinal substances in themselves; a natural pharmacopoeia; an extensive list of the specific symptoms and changes in health produced by each active medicine thus investigated, recorded in the way in which they came to the attention of the provers; disease manifestations similar (homoeopathic) to a number of natural diseases that they will one day cure—in a word, artificial disease states providing for similar natural ones the only true, homoeopathic, i.e., specific, instruments of rapid, certain, permanent cure.

   a. Lately, unknown people have been commissioned to do provings of medicines at some distance away, for the purpose of publication. But in this way the all-important work meant to be the only true basis of the art of healing and requiring the greatest moral certainty and reliability unfortunately becomes ambiguous and uncertain in its results, therefore useless. Any of the false statements to be expected from such procedures which are later accepted by homoeopathic physicians as the truth will certainly lead to most harmful consequences for patients.

144

All conjecture, everything merely asserted or entirely fabricated, must be completely excluded from such a materia medica: everything must be the pure language of nature carefully and honestly interrogated.

145

Of course, only a very extensive stock of medicines whose pure effects in altering human health are precisely known can enable us to find a suitable analogue, an artificial (curative) disease-producing power, for *every one* of the innumerable disease states in nature, for *every* chronic illness in the world.[a]

But meanwhile, even now, thanks to the reliability of symptoms and the wealth of disease manifestations already observed in each of these powerful medicinal substances in its pure effects on the healthy, there are but few cases of disease left for which a relatively suitable homoeopathic remedy cannot be found from among the medicines so far proved.[b] Such a remedy restores health easily, mildly, surely, and permanently—*infinitely* more certainly than all previous general or specialized allopathic therapies, which only alter and aggravate chronic diseases with their unknown mixed remedies and cannot cure them, which impede the cure of acute ones instead of advancing it, and which often endanger life.

a. In the beginning (some forty years ago) I was the only one for whom proving the pure powers of medicines was the most important occupation. Since that time I have been helped by a few young men who have made tests on themselves and whose observations I have examined critically. And since then some valid work in this field has been done by a few others. But what will we not be able to achieve in therapy throughout the endless field of disease when numbers of *careful and reliable* observers will have earned the merit of enriching this only true materia medica by careful *self-provings!* The healing art will then approach the mathematical sciences in certainty.

b. See footnote *a* to par. 109.

146

The *third point* of procedure [par. 72 and par. 105] for the true physician concerns the *most effective employment* of artificial disease agents whose pure action on the healthy has been proved—*medicines for the homoeopathic cure of natural diseases.*

147

Among the medicines investigated for their power to change human health, the one whose observed symptoms are most similar to the totality of symptoms of a given natural disease will be, must be, the most appropriate, the surest homoeopathic remedy for the natural disease: it is the specific for that case.

148

The natural disease must never be regarded as a noxious *substance* residing somewhere inside or outside of man (par. 11 and par. 13), but rather as something produced by a spirit-like inimical power that, as if by a kind of infection (footnote, par. 11), upsets the spirit-like vital principle in its instinctive control of the entire organism, torments it like an evil spirit, and forces it to produce in the flow of life particular sufferings and disorders called disease (symptoms).

If the vital principle is made to stop feeling the action of this inimical agent that strives to cause and perpetuate the disorder, i.e., if the physician acts on the patient with an artificial disease agent (homoeopathic medicine) that can pathologically untune the vital principle in the most similar possible way and that, even in the smallest dose, is always more energetic than the similar natural disease (par. 33 and par. 279), then during the action of this stronger similar artificial disease, that feeling of the original disease agent becomes lost to the vital principle; from that moment on the trouble no longer exists for it and is annihilated.

As we have said, if the well-chosen homoeopathic medicine is correctly used, the acute natural disease to be overcome goes away, together with all traces of sickness, imperceptibly if it is recent, often in a few hours, and if somewhat older (after employment of a few more doses of the same medicine more highly potentized or after more careful selection of some even more similar homoeopathic medicine),[a] rather later. Nothing but health and recovery follows in imperceptible, often rapid transition. The vital principle once again feels free and able to carry on the healthy life of the organism as before; vitality returns.

a. But this arduous, sometimes very arduous search and selection of the remedy in all respects homoeopathically most suitable for a given disease condition is a procedure that, despite all the commendable books facilitating it, still requires the study of the sources themselves, as well as great circumspection and serious reflection. The knowledge of having faithfully performed this duty is its best reward. Why should this difficult, careful work, the only thing that enables us to cure diseases in the best way, please these gentlemen of the new mongrel sect who boastfully claim the honorable title of homoeopath, and give for show medicines that look like homoeopathic remedies but are of course chosen only perfunctorily (*quidquid in buccam venit*)? If this incorrect medicine does not help immediately, they lay the blame not on their own unpardonable laziness and frivolity in making short work of this gravest, most important of all human concerns, but on homoeopathy, which they accuse of great imperfection (in reality the only imperfection is that the most appropriate homoeopathic remedy for every disease state does not fall into their laps without effort!). Skilled that they are, they quickly console themselves for the inefficacy of their less-than-half-homoeopathic medicines by summoning the more familiar allopathic lackey, with whom one or a few dozen leeches on the affected part, or small, innocent bloodlettings of eight ounces each, make their right regal appearance. If in spite of all this the patient survives, they extol the bloodlettings, leeches, etc., without which, they say, he would never have pulled through, and make it quite clear that these operations, borrowed without much mental effort from the ruinous routines of the old school, have in the final analysis accomplished most in the treatment. But if the patient dies, which not infrequently happens, they try to calm the inconsolate relatives by saying, "Of course you saw for yourselves that everything possible was done for the dearly departed." Who would want to honor such frivolous and pernicious rabble by calling them, after that very painstaking but beneficial art, *homoeopathic physicians?* It would serve them right to be treated in the same way when they were sick!

149

The cure of old chronic illnesses, particularly those that are complicated, requires proportionately more time. In particular, chronic medicinal diseases produced by the allopathic unhealing art, and so often coexisting with the natural diseases left uncured by it, require far more time for recovery; they are often even incurable, because of the shameless robbing of the patient's strength and vitality (from bloodlettings, purges, etc.), because of the often prolonged use of large doses of violent remedies on empty, false assumptions of their usefulness in cases that *seem* similar, and because of the prescribing of unsuitable mineral baths, etc.—"all the usual heroic deeds of allopathic so-called therapy."

150

If someone complains of one or more trifling symptoms that he has noticed only recently, the physician should not consider this a full-fledged disease requiring serious medical attention. A slight adjustment in the diet and in the mode of living usually suffices to remove this indisposition.

151

If, however, the patient complains of a few intense symptoms, the physician usually finds upon investigation several other symptoms, which, though minor, complete the picture of the disease.

152

The worse the acute disease, the more numerous and striking its symptoms usually are but the more surely can a suitable remedy be found for it if one has a sufficient number of medicines of known positive action from which to choose. Among the symptom lists of the many medicines, one can without difficulty find *one* from whose individual disease manifestations the picture of a curative artificial disease very similar to the totality of symptoms of the natural disease can be formed. This is the desired remedy.

153

In this quest for a homoeopathically specific remedy, i.e., in comparing the totality of symptoms of the natural disease with the symptom lists of available medicines so as to find a disease agent similar to the trouble being treated, the more *striking, strange, unusual, peculiar* (characteristic) signs and symptoms in the case are especially, almost exclusively, the ones to which close attention should be given, because it is *these above all which must correspond to very similar symptoms in the symptom list of the medicine being sought* if it is to be the one most suitable for cure.[a] More general and indefinite symptoms, such as loss of appetite, headache, weakness, troubled sleep, discomfort, etc., if not more precisely qualified, deserve little attention, because one finds something general of the kind in almost every disease and almost every medicine.

a. In setting out the characteristic symptoms of homoeopathic medicines in his repertory, Baron von Bönninghausen has earned our esteem, and so has Dr. G. H. G. Jahr, in his handbook *Haupt-Anzeigen,* now in its third edition under the title *Grand Manuel.*

154

If the corresponding image found in the symptom list of the nearest medicine contains in greatest number and most similarly the singular, uncommon, truly distinctive (characteristic) symptoms to be covered in the disease being treated, then *this* medicine is the most suitable one, the specific homoeopathic remedy for *this* case, and one dose of it will usually remove and extinguish a fairly recent disease, with no significant ill effects.

155

I repeat, *with no significant ill effects*. Because when this most suitable homoeopathic medicine is used, only the medicinal symptoms of the remedy which correspond to the disease symptoms act; they supplant the latter (weaker) ones in the organism, i.e., in the sensation of the vital principle, and annihilate them by exceeding them. The often very numerous remaining symptoms of the homoeopathic medicine, which are not applicable to the case at hand, remain entirely silent. Almost no trace of them can be perceived in the patient's condition, which improves by the hour, because the medicinal dose required in such high attenuation for homoeopathic use is far too weak to express in the undiseased parts of the body its remaining symptoms, the ones not similar to the case, and allows only the homoeopathic symptoms to act on the parts of the organism already very highly irritated and excited by the similar disease symptoms, so that the sick vital principle is allowed to feel only the similar but stronger medicinal disease whereby the original disease is extinguished.

156

Nevertheless, there is hardly any homoeopathic medicine, even apparently well chosen, which during its action does not bring about in very susceptible, sensitive patients *some* very slight, unaccustomed complaint or small new symptom, particularly if the dose is not attenuated enough, because it is almost impossible for the symptoms of the medicine and those of the disease to coincide as precisely as two congruent triangles. Any discrepancy, normally insignificant, is easily extinguished, however, by the inherent power (autocracy) of the living organism and does not become noticeable to patients who are not oversensitive; recovery proceeds in spite of it, if not impeded by foreign medicinal influences on the patient, or errors in living, or passions.

157

But however certain it is that a homoeopathically chosen remedy, because of its appropriateness and the minuteness of the dose, gently removes and destroys its analogous *acute* disease without manifesting its remaining unhomoeopathic symptoms, i.e., without arousing any new significant complaints, it is nevertheless usual (but only when the dose is not appropriately attentuated) for it to effect some *small* aggravation in the first hour or first few hours after it is taken and for several hours if the dose is rather too large. This aggravation is so similar to the original disease that to the patient it appears to be an aggravation of his own complaint. In fact, it is a highly similar *medicinal disease,* somewhat stronger than the original complaint.

158

This slight *homoeopathic aggravation* in the first hours is a good portent that the *acute* disease will probably be cured by the first dose and is not unusual, since the medicinal disease must naturally be somewhat

stronger than the complaint being treated to overcome
and extinguish it, just as a natural disease must be
stronger to remove and annihilate another similar one
(par. 43 to par. 48).

159

The smaller the dose of the homoeopathic remedy in
the treatment of *acute* diseases, the milder and shorter
is this apparent intensification of the disease in the first
hours.

160

But since the dose of the homoeopathic remedy can
hardly ever be so small that it cannot relieve and overcome, indeed, fully cure and destroy a recently arisen,
analogous, unspoiled natural disease (par. 249, footnotes *a* and *b*), one can understand why the right homoeopathic medicine given in a dose not as small as
possible does bring about in the first few hours a noticeable homoeopathic aggravation of this kind.[a]

a. This exaltation of the medicinal symptoms over
their analogous disease symptoms, which looks like an
aggravation, has been observed by other physicians
when they have unwittingly happened to use a homoeopathic remedy. When the scabies patient complains of
an aggravated eruption after taking sulphur, the physician consoles him with the assurance that the scabies
must completely come out before being cured, even
though he does not know why this is so; he does not
know that this is a sulphur eruption, which only looks
like an aggravation of scabies. "The facial eruption
which *Viola tricolor* cured had at first been aggra-

vated by it," as Leroy attested (*Heilk. für Mütter*, p. 406); but he did not know that the apparent aggravation came from giving this remedy, here somewhat homoeopathic, in too large a dose. Lysons said (*Med. Transact.*, London, 1772, vol. II), "Elm bark most surely cures those cutaneous eruptions which it at first aggravates." If he had given the bark, not in the monstrously large doses usual in the allopathic school, but in the very small doses needed when the medicine is prescribed on the basis of similarity of symptoms, i.e., homoeopathically, he would have cured without or almost without this apparent exacerbation of the disease (homoeopathic aggravation).

161

When I say that the so-called homoeopathic aggravation, or rather the primary action of the homoeopathic medicine, which appears to increase somewhat the symptoms of the original disease, takes place in the first hour or the first few hours, this is certainly true in more acute troubles of recent onset; but when long-acting medicines are to overcome *an old or very old chronic disease,* none of these apparent exacerbations of the original disease should be allowed to take place during the treatment. They do not appear if the accurately chosen medicine administered in appropriately small doses, which are only gradually increased, is each time somewhat modified by further dynamization (par. 247).[a] When this is done, these exacerbations of the original symptoms of the chronic disease can appear only at the end of the treatment, when the cure is complete or nearly complete.

a. If the doses of the medicine dynamized in the best way (par. 270) are small enough and if each dose is further modified in this way by shaking, then even long-acting medicines can be repeated at short intervals, even in chronic diseases.

162

Because there are still only a limited number of medicines whose true, pure effects are precisely known, it sometimes happens that only *some* of the symptoms of the disease being treated can be found in the symptom list of the medicine that is as yet the most appropriate. Such a less perfect medicinal disease agent must be used for want of a more perfect one.

163

In such cases, of course, no complete, uncomplicated cure can be expected from the medicine, because during its use a few symptoms not found earlier in the disease appear; these are side effects of a medicine that was not quite appropriate. But they do not prevent a considerable part of the trouble from being removed by the medicine—the disease symptoms that are similar to those of the medicine—nor do they hinder a good start toward cure. With appropriately small doses of the remedy, such unavoidable side effects are only mild.

164

When, however, there are only a limited number of homoeopathic symptoms to be found in the best-selected medicine, it does not prejudice the cure *if these few medicinal symptoms are for the most part uncommon ones particularly characteristic of the disease;* cure then follows with no unusual ill effects.

165

But if none of the symptoms of the medicine chosen
are exactly similar to the distinctive (characteristic), peculiar, uncommon ones of the case, and if the medicine
corresponds to the disease only in vague, general symptoms that are not more closely qualified (nausea, weakness, headache, etc.), and if no more homoeopathically
suitable medicine is to be found among those known,
then the physician should not expect any immediately
favorable outcome from the use of this unhomoeopathic
medicine.

166

Nevertheless, because today the pure effects of a
greater number of medicines are known, such a situation *very rarely* arises, and when it does, its bad consequences are mitigated as soon as an accurately similar
medicine is found to follow it.

167

In other words, if the first medicine chosen is imperfectly homoeopathic and has caused rather significant
side effects, then, in acute diseases, one does not allow
it to run its course completely and subject the patient to
the full duration of its action. One re-examines the disease condition now modified and writes down a new
disease picture consisting of the original symptoms together with the newly arisen ones.

168

Having done this, one will more easily find from
among the known medicines an analogue that corresponds to the picture and that will with the first dose

entirely destroy the disease or at least bring it much closer to cure. If this medicine is not quite enough to restore the patient's health, one continues in the same way with successive re-evaluations of the residual disease condition, selecting each time the most suitable homoeopathic medicine possible, until the complete restoration of the patient's health has been achieved.

169

If in examining a case and choosing a remedy for the first time one finds that the symptom complex of the disease is not sufficiently covered by the symptoms of any one remedy, because not enough medicines are known, and that two medicines rival each other in suitability, the first homoeopathically fitting one part of the symptoms more and the second another part, it is not advisable after giving the better of the two to resort to the other without re-evaluating the case,[a] because the medicine found in the beginning to be the second best might no longer fit the symptoms remaining under the altered circumstances.

In such cases a different remedy homoeopathically more suitable should be selected instead of the second one for the newly assessed set of symptoms.

a. And much less advisable to give both together (par. 273).

170

Therefore, here, as in all other cases where a change in the disease condition has occurred, the remaining set of symptoms must be ascertained afresh and a homoeopathic remedy as appropriate as possible to this new condition must be chosen, regardless of the medicine that previously seemed to be the second best.

If it happens that the medicine that previously seemed the second in suitability does after all prove to be appropriate to the remaining disease condition (which is rare), then it will thereby all the more merit one's confidence that it is the right one.

171

In nonvenereal chronic diseases, therefore those most usually arising from psora, one often needs to use several antipsoric remedies in succession to bring about a cure, each to be chosen because it is homoeopathic to the group of symptoms remaining after the previous one has completed its action.

172

A similar *difficulty* arises *when there are not enough symptoms in the disease being treated.* This problem deserves our careful attention because by overcoming it we have removed almost all the difficulties in this most perfect of all possible methods of healing (except that the storehouse of homoeopathically known medicines is still incomplete).

173

In the diseases that seem less amenable to cure because of an apparent paucity of symptoms, one or two symptoms predominate, obscuring almost all the others. We call them *defective diseases,* and they are usually chronic.

174

Their principal symptom can be either an internal complaint (e.g., headache or diarrhea of many years' duration, an old cardialgia, etc.) or a more external complaint. The latter are usually referred to as *local diseases*.

175

In defective illnesses of the former kind it is *often* only a matter of the medical observer's inattentiveness if he does not fully detect the symptoms that are there and that would allow him to complete the outline of the disease image.

176

Nevertheless, there certainly are a few troubles of this kind which present after all initial investigation (par. 84 to par. 98) only a few strong, intense symptoms, while the rest are indistinct.

177

Now, in order to bring such cases as *these,* which are *very rare,* to successful conclusion, one chooses to begin with, guided by these few symptoms, the medicine that is as far as one can tell the most homoeopathically suitable.

178

It certainly will sometimes happen that this medicine, chosen with scrupulous observance of homoeopathic law, will provide the appropriately similar artificial disease to annihilate the natural disease, especially if the small number of disease symptoms are very striking, definite, and peculiar or particularly distinctive (characteristic).

179

But more frequently the first medicine chosen will be only partially appropriate, for lack of a considerable number of symptoms leading to the accurate choice.

180

Here the medicine, which was chosen as well as possible but which is only incompletely homoeopathic, for the reason mentioned above, will produce side effects during its action on the disease, which is only partly analogous to it, and will admix into the economy of the patient several symptoms from its own symptom complex, as in the case above, where the selection was imperfect because of the paucity of homoeopathic remedies (par. 162). *But these symptoms are at the same time complaints belonging to the disease itself, even if they were seldom felt before, or not at all.*

Symptoms that shortly before the patient did not perceive will reveal themselves; or ones that he perceived only unclearly will become more highly developed.

181

One should not object that these side effects and new disease symptoms now apparent are to be attributed to the remedy. They come as a result of using it,[a] but they are only the symptoms that *this* disease was apt to produce by itself and in *this* organism, and the medicine merely calls them forth and brings them out by its power of producing similar ones. In a word, one has to regard the whole group of symptoms now visible as belonging to the disease itself, as its true present state, and conduct further treatment accordingly.

a. When not caused by a significant error in day-to-day living, a violent emotion, or a tumultuous change in the organism, such as the onset or cessation of menses, conception, childbirth, etc.

182

Thus the imperfect choice of a remedy, here almost inevitable because there are too few symptoms present, serves to complete the symptom content of the disease and facilitates the choice of a second, more homoeopathic medicine.

183

Therefore, as soon as the dose of the first medicine no longer has any beneficial effect (unless the newly arisen complaints require more urgent relief because of their intensity—something that is almost never the case in very chronic diseases, and because the dose of the homoeopathic medicine is so small) the case must be taken anew, recording the *status morbi* as it now is, and upon the basis of this a second homoeopathic medicine exactly suited to the present condition must be selected. It can be selected all the more accurately since the group of symptoms has become more numerous and more complete.[a]

a. When, however, the patient feels very ill although his symptoms are insignificant (something that is very rare in chronic diseases, less so in acute ones), so that the condition can be attributed more to a dulling of his nerves preventing the clear perception of his pains and complaints, opium removes this internal anesthesia, and in its secondary action the symptoms of the disease appear clearly.

184

After each medicine has completed its action, if it is found to be no longer suitable and helpful, one takes the case anew, recording the group of symptoms remaining and selecting once again the most suitable homoeopathic remedy for them, continuing in this way until the patient is cured.

185

Among defective diseases so-called *local diseases* take an important place, by which term we mean changes and complaints appearing on the external parts of the body. Until now it was taught that these parts alone were diseased, without the participation of the rest of the organism—an absurd theoretical doctrine that has led to the most ruinous medical treatment.

186

So-called *local conditions* but recently arisen and due only to external injury would at first appear to merit the name of *local diseases*. But that would be the case only if the injury were so trivial as to be without any significance, because external injuries to the body of any significance at all engage the sympathy of the whole living organism: fevers arise, etc. Such things are the proper domain of surgery only to the extent that it becomes necessary to bring help to bear on the suffering parts by mechanically removing external impediments to cure (which only the vital force can provide), e.g., by reducing dislocations, closing wounds with sutures and bandages, mechanically checking and stopping the bleeding of opened arteries, withdrawing foreign bodies that have penetrated living parts, opening a body cavity to remove a substance causing trouble or to drain extravasated or collected fluids, aligning the ends of a broken bone and securing them with proper bandaging, etc.

When in such injuries, however, the entire living organism demands effective dynamic help to be enabled to accomplish the cure, *as it always does,* when the violent fever arising from extensive contusions, from torn flesh, tendons, and vessels needs to be removed by an internal medicine or when the outer pain of a burned or excoriated part needs to be removed homoeopathically, this is where the services of the physician and his dynamic homoeopathic help come in.

187

But troubles, changes, and complaints on the external parts which have not been caused by any outer injury at all or have been precipitated by only a small one arise in an entirely different way: they arise from an inner malady. To pass them off as merely local ailments and to treat them exclusively or almost exclusively with local applications or other such means, as if they were wounds, which medicine has done through the centuries until now, is as absurd as its results are pernicious.

188

These troubles are considered to be merely local and therefore are termed *local diseases,* as if they occurred exclusively in places in which the organism took little or no part or were sufferings of individual visible parts which the rest of the living organism did not know about, as it were.[a]

a. This is one of the many pernicious absurdities of the old school.

189

And yet it is obvious even upon the slightest reflection that no external ailment not due to some particular outer injury can arise and maintain its place, or even grow worse, without inner cause, without involvement of the entire organism (which is consequently ill). They could not appear at all without the consent of all the rest of the economy and without the participation of the rest of the living whole (i.e., of the vital principle pervading all the other sensing and responsive parts of the organism). Indeed, they could not conceivably thrive without having been set in motion by the whole untuned life, so closely are all the parts of the organism interconnected, forming an indivisible whole of feeling and function. There is no lip eruption, no whitlow but the person is inwardly ill before it and while it lasts.

190

All proper medical treatment of a trouble arisen upon the external parts of the body with but little or no external injury must therefore be directed to the totality, to the annihilation and cure of the general malady through use of internal remedies if it is to be effective, sure, successful, and thorough.

191

This is categorically confirmed by experience, which shows in all cases that immediately after being taken, every active internal medicine brings about in so-called *local diseases,* even of the furthest extremities of the body, significant changes, particularly in the affected external parts (parts considered by the old school to be isolated) and in every other part of the patient's economy as well.

If the internal medicine prescribed for the totality is correctly homoeopathic, these changes will be of the most salutary kind; they are the cure of the whole man, along with the disappearance of his outer trouble (without the use of any external remedy).

192

This can best be done if when one is taking the case the exact characteristics of the local malady are considered in conjunction with all the changes, complaints, and symptoms perceptible in the rest of the patient's economy (including those noticed previously while he was not taking medicines), so as to trace out the complete disease picture before choosing, from among the remedies whose characteristic disease actions are known, the homoeopathic one corresponding to this totality of symptoms.

193

This medicine, given only internally, simultaneously removes and cures both the local disease and the concomitant disease condition in the organism, and if the trouble has only recently arisen, it often does so with the first dose. This proves that the local malady depends exclusively on a disease of the rest of the organism and is to be regarded only as an inseparable part of the whole disease, as one of its most important and striking symptoms.

194

Neither in local diseases that are acute and arise quickly nor in those that have existed for a long time is it useful to rub in or apply to the part an external remedy, not even the specific one that would be homoeopathically curative if used internally and not even if it is being used internally at the same time. This is because acute topical affections (e.g., inflammations of individual parts, erysipelas, etc.) that owe their origin, not to any external injury of proportionate violence, but to dynamic, inner causes respond most reliably (usually without other help) to internal remedies that have been chosen from the general stock of proved medicines and are homoeopathically appropriate to the inner and outer conditions of the economy evident at the time. But if these diseases do not yield to them completely and if, even though the patient is living correctly, there still remains in the suffering part and in the whole economy a residue of disease that the vital force cannot overcome, then, as is not infrequently the case, the acute local trouble is due to a flare-up of psora previously dormant within and now about to develop into an overt chronic disease.

195

In such cases, which are not infrequent, after the acute condition has been overcome as much as possible, an appropriate antipsoric treatment must be undertaken for these residual complaints and for the previous diseased state of health usual for the patient, in order to achieve a complete cure. In chronic local diseases that are not obviously venereal, the antipsoric internal cure is in any case primarily what is required.[a]

a. As I have stated in my book, *Chronic Diseases.*

196

One might think that the cure of such diseases would be accelerated if one used the remedy found to be homoeopathically correct for the totality of symptoms not only internally but externally as well, on the ground that the direct action of a medicine on the place where the disease is localized would effect a more rapid change in it.

197

But such treatment is thoroughly reprehensible, not only in local symptoms arising from the psoric miasm but also in those arising from the syphilitic or the sycotic miasm, because *to use a remedy locally at the same time as one is using it internally, in diseases that have a persistent local affection as their principal symptom,* has the serious disadvantage that, through the local application, this principal symptom (local disease)[a] usually disappears from sight before the internal disease is destroyed and thus deceives us with the appearance of a complete cure. At the least the premature disappearance of this local symptom makes it more difficult and in some cases even impossible to judge whether the whole disease has been destroyed by the simultaneous use of the internal medicine.

a. Recent scabies eruption, chancre, fig-wart.

198

For the same reason it is thoroughly reprehensible to use a remedy that has the power to cure when given internally *only* by applying it *externally* on the local symptoms of chronic miasmatic diseases. Because if the local symptom of the chronic disease is removed merely by external, defective means, one is left in the dark about the internal treatment, which is essential for the complete restoration of health. The principal symptom (the local disease) has disappeared, leaving behind only other, more indiscernible ones, which are less stable and constant than it and often are not peculiar and characteristic enough to provide a clear and complete outline of the disease picture.

199

Moreover, if the remedy homoeopathically appropriate to the disease has not yet been found at the time when the local symptom is destroyed by a caustic or desiccative external remedy or surgically,[a] the case becomes far more difficult, because the remaining symptoms are too indefinite (uncharacteristic) and fluctuating and because we can no longer see the external principal symptom, which could most of all have determined the right remedy and led us to use it internally, thus destroying the disease completely.

a. Which used to happen before I discovered the remedies for fig-wart disease (and the antipsoric medicines).

200

If it were still there during the internal treatment, one would have been able to find the homoeopathic remedy for the whole disease. Once this was found, and while it was being used only internally, the continuing presence of the local disease would indicate that the cure was not yet complete; on the other hand, if the local disease healed without any suppressive external interference, this would indicate incontrovertibly that the trouble had been rooted out and that the desired cure of the whole disease had been accomplished—so it is an inestimable, indispensable help in the achievement of complete cure.

201

It seems that when burdened with a chronic disease that it cannot overcome by its own means, the vital force decides (instinctively) to form a local disease on some external part, with the exclusive object of allaying the internal disease, which would otherwise threaten the vital organs and life. It creates and maintains a disease on an external part not essential to life, as it were diverting and consigning the internal disease to a vicarious local one. In this way the local disease silences the internal disease for a time, but without being able to heal or materially diminish it.[a]

The local disease is never anything but a part of the disease totality, but it is a part disproportionately developed by the organic vital force and transferred to a less dangerous (external) part of the body in order to allay the internal disease.

As we have said, the vital force accomplishes so little toward reducing or curing the whole disease through this local symptom that silences it that, on the contrary, the internal disease gradually increases, and nature has to enlarge and aggravate the local symptom more and more for it to continue serving as a substitute that allays the growing internal disease. Old leg ulcers become worse in uncured internal psora, the chancre increases in uncured syphilis, fig-warts multiply and grow in uncured sycosis, which becomes more and more difficult to cure, as the whole internal disease grows by itself with time.

a. The fontanels of the old school physicians have a similar effect. These artificial ulcers on an external part allay some internal chronic complaints, but only for a very short time (for as long as they produce in the diseased organism an unaccustomed painful irritation), and are not able to cure them; instead they weaken and ruin the entire economy far more than the instinctive vital force does with most of its metastases.

202

If the physician of the old school destroys the local symptom by some external means, thinking thereby to heal the entire disease, nature compensates for this by awakening the internal malady and the other symptoms that have lain dormant next to the local disease all along, i.e., it increases the internal disease. In such cases one usually says, *incorrectly,* that the local disease has been *driven back* into the body or upon the nerves by external means.

203

Any external treatment to remove such local symptoms from the surface of the body without having cured the internal miasmatic disease—e.g., removing scabies eruption with all kinds of ointments, burning away the chancre with caustics, destroying fig-warts only by cutting, tying, or cauterizing—all such pernicious external treatment, up to now so widespread, has become the most common source of the innumerable chronic ailments with and without names under which mankind so universally groans. It is one of the greatest crimes the medical fraternity could commit, and yet up to now it has been the generally established procedure, and the universities have been teaching that it is the only one.[a]

a. Because any medicines that they might give in addition to this external treatment only aggravate the disease, since their remedies have no specific curative power for the disease totality but certainly do attack and weaken the organism and inflict other chronic medicinal diseases on it.

204

Apart from all the chronic troubles, complaints, and diseases arising from a prolonged unhealthy way of living (par. 77) and the innumerable chronic medicinal diseases (par. 74) arising from the unwise, persistent, violent, and pernicious treatment that the old school employs, often even for minor complaints, most chronic diseases develop from these three chronic miasms: internal syphilis, internal sycosis, but most of all, and to a disproportionate extent, internal psora.

Each of these miasms has already occupied the entire organism and permeated all its parts before the appearance of the primary, vicarious local symptom (the scabies eruption in psora, the chancre or inguinal bubo in syphilis, and the fig-warts in sycosis), which prevents its full manifestation.

If these miasms are by external means deprived of the vicarious local symptoms that allay the general internal malady, sooner or later the characteristic diseases that the Creator of nature has decreed for each of them must inevitably develop and manifest fully and thus spread all the nameless misery, the incredible multitude of chronic diseases, which have plagued the human race for hundreds and thousands of years.

None of them would have manifested themselves so often if physicians had wisely endeavored to cure these three miasms fundamentally and to extinguish them in the organism exclusively by the internal use of homoeopathic medicines appropriate to each, without disturbing their external symptoms through topical treatment (footnote, par. 282).

205

The homoeopathic physician never treats any of these primary symptoms of chronic miasms or any of the secondary ones arising during their development by local means (neither with external dynamically acting ones nor with mechanical ones).[a] He cures only the great underlying miasm instead, whereupon its primary (except in some cases of long-standing sycosis) and secondary symptoms spontaneously disappear as well. But since this is never the method of treatment which has been followed before the homoeopathic physician comes upon the scene, he usually finds that the primary symptoms[b] have regrettably already been destroyed externally by previous physicians, and he now has to deal more with the secondary ones, i.e., the ones arising from the full manifestation and development of the indwelling miasms—most often with the chronic diseases of internal psora. In my book on the chronic diseases, to which I here refer the reader, I have presented the internal cure of these miasms as thoroughly as any one physician could do after many years of reflection, observation, and experience.

a. Therefore I cannot, for example, advise that so-called labial or facial cancer (a product, perhaps, of advanced psora, not infrequently combined with syphilis) should be locally extirpated with Cosmo's arsenical preparation, not only because this treatment is extremely painful and frequently fails but especially because when it does remove the malignant ulcer from the place, the fundamental malady has not in the least been diminished; the life-preserving force has therefore to displace the focus of the general internal disease to a more important part of the organism (as it does in all metastases), so that blindness, deafness, insanity, asthma, dropsy, apoplexy, etc., follow. Moreover, this dubious procedure of removing the local malignant ulcer with the topical arsenical preparation succeeds only when the ulcer is not too large, and when it is not syphilitic, and when the vital force is still very energetic; but it is precisely in such cases that the complete internal cure of the whole underlying disease is still possible.

Similar results occur if, without the previous cure of the indwelling miasm, facial or breast cancer is removed only surgically or encysted tumors are enucleated. Something worse follows; at the least death comes more quickly. This has happened in innumerable cases, yet in each new case the old school still blindly continues to inflict the same misery.

b. Scabies eruption, chancre (inguinal bubo), fig-warts.

206

Before starting the treatment of a chronic disease the physician must most scrupulously inquire whether the patient has had a syphilitic infection (or fig-wart gonorrhea).[a] If he has, it is *this* that must be treated, and if the symptoms are exclusively those of syphilis (or of the rarer fig-wart disease), only this—but in recent times such pure cases have been very rare. In any case of psora with a previous history of such an infection, the latter must be taken into consideration, because it will have complicated the psora. This is always what has happened when there are venereal symptoms that are not pure.

When the physician believes that he has an old case of syphilis before him, it is always, or almost always, one that is combined (complicated) mainly with psora, because the internal chronic scabies disease (psora) is by far the *most frequent underlying cause of chronic diseases*. Sometimes he will be confronted with both these miasms, further complicated with sycosis, in chronic cases that have had the latter infection. But far more frequently, psora alone is the fundamental cause of all the other chronic complaints (whatever name they might bear), complaints that have usually been exacerbated and monstrously distorted by previous allopathic bungling.

a. In such inquiries one should not be misled by the more common explanations of patients or relatives, who attribute the origin of chronic diseases, even the gravest, most inveterate ones, either to the catching of a cold many years before (from becoming wet or taking a cold drink when heated), or to a fright, or to lifting a heavy weight, or to a violent emotion (even perhaps to witchcraft), etc. Such things are far too insignificant to produce a chronic disease *in a healthy person*, to sustain it for many years, and to make it grow from year to year, as happens in all chronic diseases belonging to developed psora. Far more important causes than these recollected mishaps must underlie the commencement and continuation of a significant inveterate complaint. Such alleged exciting causes can only indicate the moment when a chronic miasm was awakened.

207

After obtaining the above information the homoeopathic physician still has to inquire into the previous allopathic treatments that the chronically ill patient has had—the principal and most frequent medicines that have interfered with the case, the mineral baths, and their results—so as to understand to some degree the degeneration of the original disease condition and as much as possible correct this artificial deterioration or at least avoid the medicines already abused.

208

After that the patient's age, way of living, diet, activities, domestic situation, social circumstances, etc., must be considered, to ascertain whether these things aggravate his trouble and to what degree they might help or interfere with the treatment. Similarly, one should not overlook his emotional and mental disposition, to ascertain whether it might be an impediment to the treatment and whether psychological attention might be necessary to guide, encourage, or change it.

209

Only then should the physician, in repeated conversations with the patient, endeavor to trace out his disease picture as completely as possible, in the manner indicated above, so as to record the most striking, most peculiar (characteristic) symptoms. On this information he starts the treatment by selecting the first (antipsoric, etc.) remedy, according to the greatest possible symptom similarity.

210

To psora belong almost all those diseases that I have termed defective and that, because they are defective, appear more difficult to cure—diseases in which all the other symptoms are, as it were, hidden behind a single, principal, predominating one. The so-called *emotional and mental diseases* are like this. But they do not constitute a class of diseases completely separate from all others, because even in so-called physical diseases the emotional and mental state is *always* affected.[a] In all diseases being treated, the psychic condition of the patient should be written down among the totality of symptoms as one of the most important, if one desires to have a faithful picture of the disease from which to make a successful homoeopathic cure.

a. For example, how often does not one find, in the most painful diseases of many years' standing, a mild, gentle disposition commanding the physician's tender consideration and compassion? But when he overcomes the disease and restores the patient, as frequently happens under homoeopathic treatment, he is often surprised and shocked at the dreadful change in the patient's nature: ingratitude, hardheartedness, unusual maliciousness, and a disposition most disgraceful and degrading to mankind often make their appearance. These are exactly the qualities that this patient had before he became ill.

One often finds that people who were patient when they were healthy become obstinate, violent, hasty, or unbearable and self-willed—indeed, impatient or despairing—when they are ill; those who were discreet and modest become obscene and shameless; those who were clearheaded become dull-witted; those who were inclined to be feebleminded seem to become rather clever and more sensible; those who were slow to decide acquire great presence of mind and decisiveness; etc.

211

This is so important that the psychic condition of the patient is often the decisive factor in choosing a homoeopathic remedy, because it is a particularly characteristic symptom and one that can least of all remain hidden from the carefully observant physician.

212

The Creator of healing forces has also made special provision for this principal aspect of all diseases, the altered emotional and mental state, because there is no potent medicinal substance in the world which does not very markedly alter the emotional and mental state of a healthy man testing it, and each medicine does this in its own distinctive way.

213

Therefore one will never cure according to nature—that is, homoeopathically—unless one considers the mental and emotional changes along with the other symptoms in all cases of disease, even acute ones, and unless for treatment one chooses from among the remedies a disease agent that can produce an emotional or mental state *of its own* similar to that of the disease[a] as well as other symptoms similar to those of the disease.

a. Thus *Aconitum napellus* will seldom or *never* cure either quickly or permanently if the disposition is calm and undisturbed; nor will *Nux vomica* if it is mild and phlegmatic; nor will *Pulsatilla* if it is glad, cheerful, and willful; nor will *Ignatia* if it is steady and without fearfulness or irritability.

214

What I have to teach about the cure of mental and emotional diseases comes down to very little: they are to be cured in exactly the same way as all other diseases, not differently, i.e., with a remedy, a disease agent capable of producing in the body and psyche of healthy people symptoms as similar as possible to those of the case.

215

Almost all so-called mental and emotional diseases are nothing but physical diseases in which the symptom of mental and emotional disorder characteristic of each one increases more or less rapidly as the physical symptoms diminish, until the disease finally attains the most striking state of defectiveness, almost like a local disease transferred into the invisibly subtle mental or emotional organs.

216

There are many cases in which a life-threatening so-called physical disease—suppuration of the lungs, or the destruction of some other vital organ, or some other violent (acute) malady (e.g., during confinement, etc.)—deteriorates into insanity or some kind of melancholy or mania through the rapid increase of the psychic symptom and thereby completely removes the threat to life occasioned by the physical symptoms, which improve during this time almost to the point of health or, rather, until their obscure continued presence can be discerned only by a physician who observes persistently and closely. In this way the cases degenerate into a defective, as it were, local disease, in which the psychic symptom, previously only mild, has grown to become the main symptom, which very largely supplants the other (physical) ones and palliatively allays their violence; in a word, the affection of the coarser physical organs is, as it were, transferred and diverted to the almost spiritual mental and emotional organs, which lie forever beyond the reach of the dissecting scalpel.

217

In these cases the physician must carefully investigate the symptom totality, primarily of course to understand exactly the particular character of the principal symptom—the specific mental and emotional state predominating in each case—but also to uncover the physical symptoms, so as to find from among the remedies whose pure effects are known a homoeopathic medicinal disease agent to extinguish the disease totality, a remedy that contains among its symptoms to the greatest possible degree of similarity not only the physical symptoms of the case but also, above all, its mental and emotional state.

218

The first thing that belongs in the symptom picture of these diseases is a precise description of all the symptoms of the previous so-called physical disease before it degenerated into a mental or emotional disease by the disproportionate growth of the mental symptom. This can be learned from the reports of the relatives.

219

The continuing veiled presence of these earlier physical symptoms is confirmed by the fact that vestiges of them remain, vestiges that are not obvious but that stand out in lucid moments when the mental disease temporarily subsides.

220

If one adds to these symptoms the mental and emotional state, accurately observed by the relatives and by the physician himself,[a] one has constituted a complete disease picture for which a medicine capable of producing exactly similar symptoms, and particularly a similar mental disturbance, can be chosen from among the (antipsoric, etc.) remedies, so that the disease may be cured homoeopathically. This is the way we proceed when the mental disease has lasted for some time.

[a]. It often appears to alternate periodically, e.g., after several days of violent insanity or rage, other days of silent melancholic depression follow, etc., or perhaps the condition returns only during certain months of the year.

221

If, however, insanity or mania (precipitated by fright, vexation, alcohol, etc.) suddenly bursts forth as an acute disease from the patient's usually calm condition, although it almost always arises from internal psora (like a flame flaring up from it), at this initial, acute stage it should immediately be treated, not with antipsoric remedies, but with medicines such as *Aconite, Belladonna, Stramonium, Hyoscyamus, Mercury,* etc., chosen from the other group of proved remedies and given in highly potentized subtle homoeopathic doses, so as to overcome it to the point where the psora returns for the time being to its former, almost latent condition, in which the patient appears to be well.

222

But such a patient delivered from an acute mental or emotional disease by these apsoric remedies should never be considered to be cured; on the contrary, one should lose no time in freeing him completely with sustained antipsoric (perhaps also antisyphilitic) treatment from the chronic miasm of the psora,[a] which is now once again dormant but very liable to recur in attacks of the same mental or emotional disease. After this no similar future attacks need be feared, on condition that the patient observes the regimen prescribed for him.

a. It is very rare for a mental or emotional disease that is already somewhat chronic to subside spontaneously (for the internal chronic disease to return to the coarser physical organs). It occasionally happens, as when an inmate of a mental institution is discharged as being apparently cured. Otherwise all mental institutions have until now remained crammed to capacity, so that the host of mental patients awaiting admission almost never find an opening unless somebody dies. *Not one of the inmates there is truly and permanently cured by the old school!* This is a convincing proof (among many others) of the complete uselessness of the unhealing art of the old school, which, ridiculously enough, the allopaths boastfully honor by calling it *rational medicine*. On the other hand, how often the true art of healing (genuine, pure homoeopathy) has restored to these unfortunate people their mental and physical health and returned them to their kin and to the world!

223

But without the antipsoric (perhaps also antisyphilitic) treatment, one may almost certainly expect an early, more persistent, more serious new attack of insanity, set off by an exciting cause even more slight than that which caused the first attack. During this new attack, the psora usually attains its complete development and turns into a periodic or continuous mental disturbance more difficult to cure antipsorically.

224

If the mental disease is not yet fully developed and if there is still some doubt whether it really has come from a physical disease or from bad upbringing, bad habits, perverted morals, lack of mental discipline, superstition, or ignorance, the following will help one to decide.

In the latter case it will diminish and improve from understanding, well-intentioned exhortations, consoling arguments, earnest and sensible explanations. On the other hand, a real emotional or mental disease due to a physical disease is quickly aggravated by such an approach: melancholia becomes more profound, plaintive, inconsolate, and withdrawn; malicious insanity becomes more spiteful; foolish chatter becomes noticeably more silly.[a]

a. It would appear here that the soul of the patient feels upset and sorrowful at the truth of this reasonable advice and acts on the body as if it wants to restore the harmony that has been lost; but the body in its disease reacts too strongly upon the mental and emotional organs, throwing them into an even greater tumult by once more transferring its sufferings back upon them.

225

Conversely, as we have said, there are of course a few psychic diseases that have not merely degenerated from physical ones; instead, with only slight physical illness, they arise and proceed from the psyche, from persistent grief, resentment, anger, humiliation, and repeated exposure to fear and fright. In time such psychic diseases often greatly harm the physical health.

226

Only these emotional diseases that come into being and are sustained through the mind *and only those that are still recent and have not yet impaired physical health too much* can be transformed speedily into psychic well-being by psychological means such as kindness, friendly exhortation, and appeal to reason, and often also by a skillful deception. In these cases, with the right living habits, physical well-being appears to follow as well.

227

The psoric miasm, however, underlies these diseases as well; it is just not yet near its full development. To make sure that the patient does not relapse into a similar mental disease, which could happen all too easily, the physician should give him thorough antipsoric (also perhaps antisyphilitic) treatment.

228

In mental and emotional diseases that arise from physical disease and that can be cured only by homoeopathic remedies for the internal miasm (along with carefully regulated living habits), the relatives and the physician must of course also carefully maintain the right psychological attitude toward the patient, surrounding him with emotional support. They must meet raving madness with calm fearlessness and firm, cool determination; agonized lamentation with mute compassion in countenance and bearing; senseless babbling with silence that is not completely indifferent; loathsome, disgusting behavior and speech with complete inattention. They must take measures to prevent damage to property, *without reproaching the patient about this,* and arrange everything in such a way that corporal punishment and torture are completely eliminated.[a]

The administration of medicines is the only thing for which one might be able to justify the use of force, but in homoeopathy this is made easier by the fact that the small doses needed to cure are *never* noticeable to the taste and can therefore be given to the patient in his drink, completely without his knowledge, making all force unnecessary.

a. The hardhearted mindlessness of physicians in many institutions of this kind is astonishing; without searching for the only right way of curing such diseases in the homoeopathic *medicinal* (antipsoric) method, the only one that works, they have the inhumanity to torment these most pathetic patients with violent beatings and other agonizing tortures. By this unconscionable and disgraceful behavior they debase themselves far below the level of prison guards, who carry out such punishment on criminals only because it is their duty. These people, on the other hand, humiliated by feelings of their own medical inaptitude, seem to vent their spite at the presumed incurability of mental and emotional diseases by displaying cruelty to the pathetic, innocent sufferers themselves. They are too ignorant to help and too lazy to adopt a therapy that works.

229

On the other hand, contradiction, ready agreement, severe reproval, insults, weakness, and timid acquiescence are all entirely inappropriate, all equally harmful to the mind and spirit of such people. But they are embittered, and their disease is aggravated most of all by scorn, deceit, and transparent deceptions.

The physician and the attendants must always behave as if they believed such patients to be sane.

One should try to remove everything external which bothers their senses or feelings. There is no diversion for their beclouded minds, no healthy amusement, no edification, no way through word or book or any other thing to soothe their souls languishing or raging in the fetters of a diseased body, no way to quicken their spirits but with cure. Not until their physical health is improved do peace and comfort shine once more upon their spirit.[a]

a. The cure of insane, raving, and melancholic patients can be accomplished only in an institution expressly appointed to that end, and not at home with their families.

230

For any particular case of mental or emotional disease (and they are incredibly varied), if the remedies chosen are in complete homoeopathic correspondence with a faithfully drawn disease picture, the smallest possible doses are often sufficient to bring about the most striking improvement quite quickly.

This is never accomplished with the massive, frequent doses of all the other inappropriate (allopathic) medicines, used until they kill the patient.

If there is a sufficiently large choice of homoeopathic medicines whose pure effects are known, the tireless search for the most suitable one becomes easier in these cases because of the fact that their principal symptom, the emotional and mental condition, manifests itself with unmistakable clarity.

Indeed, from much experience I can state that the great superiority of homoeopathy over every other conceivable therapy is nowhere so triumphantly revealed as in inveterate emotional and mental diseases arising from a physical disease or along with it.

231

We must now consider *intermittent diseases,* not only those that recur at definite intervals, such as the large number of intermittent fevers and apparently nonfebrile recurrent complaints, but also those in which particular disease conditions alternate with others of a different nature at indefinite intervals.

232

The latter, the *alternating diseases,* are also very numerous.[a] But they all belong to the chronic diseases;

they are usually a product of developed psora by itself, only rarely complicated with a syphilitic miasm. In the first case therefore they are to be treated with antipsoric remedies and in the second case with antipsoric remedies alternating with antisyphilitic ones, as explained in my book on the chronic diseases.

a. Two or even three different states can succeed each other: e.g., in twofold alternating diseases it can happen that continuous pains in the feet, etc., appear as soon as inflammation of the eye subsides and that the latter reasserts itself as soon as the pain in the extremities subsides; spasms and convulsions can alternate immediately with any other complaint of the body or of a part of it; and in threefold cyclic diseases one might find, in the midst of continual sickliness, sudden periods of apparent well-being and a strained increase in mental and physical powers (exaggerated mirthfulness, an overagitated physical liveliness, an excessive sense of well-being, immoderate appetite, etc.), followed by an equally sudden gloomy, melancholic mood, an unbearable hypochondriacal emotional state, with disturbances of many vital functions such as digestion, sleep, etc., followed in turn and just as suddenly by the accustomed malaise. Similar things happen in many other cyclic diseases with multiple phases. Often no trace of the previous phase can be noticed when the new one appears; in other cases a few symptoms of the previous state remain during the commencement and continuation of the next. Sometimes the successive morbid states are completely opposite in nature, e.g., melancholia periodically alternating with gay insanity or frenzy.

233

The *intermittent diseases* are ones in which the same disease condition returns at fairly definite intervals in the midst of apparent well-being and leaves after an equally definite period. One finds this both in apparently nonfebrile conditions that nevertheless come and go at definite intervals and in febrile ones—the various intermittent fevers—as well.

234

The apparently nonfebrile disease states mentioned, which recur at definite intervals in a single patient (they do not usually occur sporadically or epidemically), always belong to the chronic diseases (for the most part purely psoric, only seldom complicated with syphilis), and they can be treated successfully as such.

Sometimes, however, the intercurrent use of a very small dose of potentized cinchona bark solution is necessary to extinguish the periodicity of the disease completely.

235

Regarding *intermittent fevers* that are sporadic or epidemic (not those endemic to marshy areas),[a] we often find that each paroxysm likewise consists of two alternating phases opposite to each other (cold-heat, heat-cold), but even more often that it consists of three phases (cold-heat-sweat). Therefore the remedy for these, chosen from among the group of proved remedies (usually not antipsorics), must ideally be able to produce both or all three successive states in a healthy person in a similar way or at least correspond as homoeopathically as possible to the strongest and most characteristic of the successive states—the cold, or the heat, or the sweat—with its accessory symptoms.

Nevertheless, the choice of the most accurate homoeopathic remedy must above all be determined by the symptoms that the patient has outside of his attacks.[b]

a. Until now, orthodox pathology, still in its irrational infancy, has recognized only a single *intermittent fever,* which it also calls *ague,* and it makes no distinctions other than the intervals at which the attacks recur (quotidian, tertian, quartan, etc.). There are, however, far more significant distinctions among these fevers than their intervals of recurrence. There are innumerable different kinds of these fevers: many of them cannot be called *agues* at all, because their paroxysms consist only of heat; others are characterized only by cold, with or without sweat afterwards; in others the patient is objectively cold all over but has a sensation of heat, or is objectively hot while experiencing chill; in others one paroxysm consists only of rigor or simple chilliness followed by a feeling of well-being, while the next consists only of heat, with or without subsequent sweat; in others the heat comes first and the chill only later; in others, after a cold and hot stage, apyrexia follows, and in a second attack, often many hours later, there is sweat alone; in others there is no sweat at all, or only sweat, without heat or chill, or sweat only during the heat. There are innumerable other distinctions to be made, primarily in the accessory symptoms—a particular kind of headache, bad taste, nausea, vomiting, diarrhea, excessive thirst or thirstlessness, particular pains of limb or abdomen, disturbances of sleep, delirium, affective disorders, convulsions, etc.—all of them coming before, during, or after the cold, the heat, the sweat. All these are obviously intermittent fevers of very different kinds, and *obviously* each one requires its own (homoeopathic) treatment.

It is true that almost every one of these can be suppressed (as so often happens) by monstrously large doses of cinchona bark or its derivative, quinine sulphate: the quinine extinguishes the periodicity, but patients with intermittent fevers for which cinchona bark is not indicated (like all those intermittent fevers that epidemically invade whole regions, even mountainous ones) are not cured when this periodicity is extinguished. On the contrary! They are only sick in a different way, often much more sick than before, from the particular chronic disease caused by cinchona, which as a rule can hardly be eradicated even after long treatment with the true art of healing. Is this their idea of *cure?*

b. Baron von Bönninghausen was the first to elucidate in the best way this subject, which needs so much circumspection, and to facilitate the selection of the remedy for these different epidemic fevers, in his work *Versuch einer homöopathischen Therapie der Wechselfieber,* Münster, Regensberg, 1833.

236

In such cases the medicine is most helpful and effective if given immediately after, or at least very soon after, the end of a paroxysm, when the patient has somewhat recovered from the attack. In this way the remedy has time to bring about all the curative changes in the organism it can, without turmoil or violence.

On the other hand, if a medicine is given immediately before a paroxysm, no matter how specifically it may be indicated, its action coincides with the new attack and sets off such a reaction, such a violent opposition in the organism, as to constitute an assault, which at the least spends much of the patient's strength, if it does not actually endanger his life.[a]

But if one gives the medicine immediately after the end of the paroxysm, that is, at the beginning of the time when the patient is most free of the fever, and well before the inception of the following attack, the vital force is in the best possible condition to be cured by the remedy in a gentle way.

a. One sees this in cases—not entirely infrequent— in which a moderate dose of opium given during the rigor has quickly ended in death.

237

But if the interval between the paroxysms is very short, as occurs in some very grave fevers, or if it is obscured by vestiges of the previous attack, the homoeopathic remedy must be given when the sweating or the last symptoms of the paroxysm that is ending begin to subside.

238

Quite frequently, the appropriate medicine wipes out several attacks with a single small dose and may even be sufficient to restore health. But in most cases one must give a new dose after each attack. In the favorable circumstance that the nature of the symptoms has not changed, this will be the same medicine. The recent discovery of the best method of repeating doses makes it possible to do this without ill effects (footnotes, par. 270). Each successive dose is dynamized by ten or twelve succussions of the bottle containing the medicinal solution.

Nevertheless, the intermittent fever sometimes (though seldom) returns after the patient has felt well for several days. But this recurrence of the same fever after an interval of health is possible only if the disease agent that first caused the intermittent fever has been reasserting its influence on the convalescent continually, as happens in marshy districts. In such cases a permanent cure is often possible only by the removal of this exciting cause (as by a sojourn in the mountains, if it is a case of marsh fever).

239

Since almost every medicine produces in its pure effects its own particular fever (even a kind of intermittent fever, with its successive phases) different from the fevers of all others, there are in the great realm of medicines homoeopathic remedies for the numerous natural intermittent fevers, and remedies for many of them can even now be found among the moderate number of remedies that have already been proved on the healthy.

240

But if the remedy found to be homoeopathically specific for a prevailing epidemic of intermittent fever does not effect a perfect cure in some patient and if the cure has not been prevented by his living in a marshy area, this always means that the psoric miasm is in the background and that antipsoric medicines must be employed until complete cure is achieved.

241

Epidemics of intermittent fevers occurring outside of places where intermittent fevers are endemic have the nature of chronic diseases, composed of individual acute attacks. Each individual epidemic has its own consistent nature common to all individuals affected. If this is established from the totality of symptoms common to all the patients, it reveals the right homoeopathic remedy, the one specific to the epidemic; this remedy almost always helps patients who were fairly healthy before the epidemic and not chronically sick with developed psora.

242

If in such an epidemic of intermittent fever, the first attacks have been left uncured, or if the patients have been weakened by allopathic mistreatment, then the psora, unfortunately inhabiting so many people, albeit latently, develops and takes on the periodicity and in all appearances plays out the role of this epidemic intermittent fever, so that the medicine that would have been useful in the initial paroxysms is no longer suitable and cannot help. We now have a case of psoric intermittent fever only; it is usually overcome by very minute doses of *Sulphur* and *Hepar sulphuris* in high potency.

243

In those often very pernicious intermittent fevers befalling single individuals outside of marshy regions, one must (as in acute diseases generally, which they resemble for their psoric origin) of course *start* treatment by using for several days a remedy homoeopathically chosen for the particular case from among the other (not antipsoric) group of proved medicines, until it has helped as much as it can. But if after this the recovery is not complete, it means that one has a case of psora about to become manifest and that only antipsoric medicines can help fundamentally.

244

Intermittent fevers endemic to marshy regions and to places where flooding is frequent have given the old school much to do. But a young person who is healthy can become accustomed even to such surroundings and stay healthy, provided that his way of living is exactly right and that he is not weighed down by deprivation, hard labor, or destructive passions; at least, intermittent fevers endemic to such places will take hold of him only if he is a newcomer, but then one or two of the *most minute* doses of highly potentized cinchona bark solution and the orderly way of life mentioned will quickly free him.

But if people cannot be freed of the marsh fevers by a few such small doses of cinchona, along with proper exercise and healthy mental and physical discipline, it always means that psora striving to manifest itself underlies their condition and that their intermittent fevers cannot be cured in the marshy area without antipsoric treatment.[a]

If they are not yet too deeply ill, i.e., if the psora has not yet completely developed in them and can therefore return to its latent state, these patients sometimes seem to recover if they promptly leave the marshy area for a dry mountainous region—the fever goes away. But they will never become really healthy without antipsoric treatment.

a. Larger, frequently repeated doses of cinchona bark, as also a concentrated cinchona preparation such as quinine sulphate, can of course relieve such patients of the periodicity typical of marsh fever, but people thus deceived into believing that they are cured continue to suffer in a different way from a quinine cachexia, which is sometimes incurable (footnote *b* to par. 276).

245

Having seen the attention that one should give in homoeopathic treatment to the principal varieties of disease and to the particular circumstances within each variety, we now pass on to the subject of *remedies: the method of using them and the regimen to be observed when taking them.*

246

As long as there is a marked, obviously progressing improvement during treatment, no more medicine of any kind must be given, because all the good that the medicine taken can accomplish is speeding toward its completion.

This is not infrequently the case with acute diseases.

If the disease is somewhat chronic, however, a single dose of the appropriately chosen homoeopathic medicine does sometimes complete the good that that remedy can according to its nature accomplish in the case, but slowly, over a period of 40, 50, 60, or 100 days. Now, for one thing, this is very rarely the case, and, secondly, it must be a matter of great importance to the physician and to the patient to reduce this period by half or three-quarters or more, if possible, so as to obtain a far more rapid cure.

As the most recent and frequently verified experiments have taught me, this can be accomplished very felicitously if the following conditions are fulfilled: firstly, if the medicine is very carefully selected so that it is accurately homoeopathic; secondly, if it is highly potentized, dissolved in water, and given in suitably small doses at intervals that experience has shown to be the most appropriate for the speediest possible cure. *But the degree of potency of each dose must be somewhat different from that of the previous and that of the following dose,* so that the vital principle, which is to be diverted to a similar medicinal disease, is never roused and incited to untoward reactions, as always happens when unmodified doses are repeated, especially at short intervals.[a]

a. What I said in the fifth edition of the *Organon* in a long footnote to this paragraph, with the purpose of preventing these untoward reactions of the vital force, was all that my experience permitted me to say at the time. But for the last four or five years thanks to the modifications by which I have perfected previous procedures, all these difficulties have been completely removed. The same well-chosen medicine can now be given daily, even for months if necessary. In the treatment of chronic diseases, if the lower degree of potency is used up in one or two weeks, one proceeds in a similar way to the higher degree. (In the new method of dynamization, to be explained later, the medicine is administered beginning with the lowest degrees.)

247

It is inadmissible to repeat, even once, exactly the same dose of medicine without modifying it,[a] let alone many times (and at short intervals, because one does not want the cure to be delayed).

The vital principle does not accept such *identical* doses without opposition, i.e., without bringing out other symptoms of the medicine, symptoms not similar to those of the disease being treated. The previous dose has already completed the transformation of the vital principle expected of it, and a second, unmodified dose of the same medicine identical in degree of dynamization is consequently no longer able to work exactly the same effect upon the vital principle. Now the patient can only be made sick in a different way by such an *unaltered* dose, basically more sick than before, because now the only symptoms left to act are the medicinal ones that are not homoeopathic to the disease. Therefore no progress toward cure but only a real aggravation of the case can result.

But if one slightly modifies the potency of each new dose by dynamizing it to a somewhat higher degree (par. 269 and par. 270), the sick vital principle allows itself to be altered further by the same medicine without ill effect (to have its awareness of the natural disease further reduced) and thereby to be brought nearer to cure.

a. This is why one should not give the patient soon afterward a second or a third dose of even the best chosen homoeopathic medicine dry, e.g., another globule of the same degree of potency which helped so much the first time. And this is also why if the remedy that has helped so much the first time is in aqueous solution, to give the patient a second or third dose, of the same amount or less, from the bottle *without shaking it* will not help him again, even if the doses are some days apart. It makes no difference whether the original preparation has been potentized with ten succussions or—according to a more recent suggestion of mine for avoiding the ill effects mentioned above—only two. And the reason for this has already been explained above.

But when each dose is modified in its degree of dynamization, as I explain here, then the doses are not a shock to the organism, even if they are repeated frequently, no matter how highly the medicine is potentized, with however many succussions. One might almost say that even the most perfectly chosen homoeopathic medicine can remove and extinguish the pathological disturbance of the vital principle in chronic diseases in the best possible way only *if it is used in several different forms.*

248

For this purpose the medicinal solution is potentized anew *each time before it is taken* (with about eight, ten, or twelve succussions of the bottle).[a] The patient should take one or (increasing progressively) more coffee spoons or teaspoons of this as follows: in chronic diseases, daily or every other day; in acute diseases, every six, four, three, or two hours; and in the most urgent cases every hour or more frequently still. In chronic diseases every correctly chosen homoeopathic medicine, even one of a long-acting nature, can be repeated daily for months in this way with ever-increasing benefit. If the solution is used up (in a week or two) one employs for the next solution of the same medicine, if it is still indicated, one or (rarely) several globules of a different (higher) degree of potency.

One proceeds in this way as long as the patient continues to feel steady improvement and does not experience any significant symptom that he has never had before. Because if he does experience new symptoms, if the disease still remaining manifests in the midst of a group of *new, different* symptoms, *then another medicine, now more homoeopathically appropriate, must be chosen in the place of the last one and likewise be administered in repeated doses*—of course always in the manner described above, i.e., never without the solution being somewhat modified before each dose with the necessary strong succussions to alter and slightly increase its degree of potency.

But if *so-called homoeopathic aggravations* (par. 161) appear toward the end of treatment in a chronic disease after the almost daily repetition of exactly the right homoeopathic medicine, i.e., if the disease symptoms remaining seem to be somewhat worse again (because the medicinal disease so similar to the natural disease is now almost the only one acting), then the doses must be reduced further and repeated at longer intervals or else stopped altogether for several days to see whether perhaps no more medicine is necessary for cure, in which case these seeming symptoms, caused only by an excess of the homoeopathic medicine, will disappear by themselves, leaving unclouded health in their wake.

If one is using in the treatment a single small vial in which a globule of the remedy has been dissolved and shaken into about a drachm of diluted wine spirit* for inhalation daily or every two, three, or four days, then this must still be strongly shaken ten or twelve times before each use.

a. This solution is prepared with forty, thirty, twenty, fifteen, or eight tablespoons of water, with the addition of a little wine spirit or a piece of charcoal to prevent the solution from spoiling. If one uses the charcoal, one hangs it in the bottle from a thread and draws it out each time the bottle has to be shaken.

Instead of dissolving the medicinal globule (one rarely needs more than a single globule of appropriately dynamized medicine) in a large amount of water, one can dissolve it in, for example, only seven or eight tablespoons of water, *shake the bottle vigorously,* pour a tablespoon of this into a drinking glass containing eight to ten tablespoons of water, *stir this vigorously,* and give the patient a specific dose of it.

*[I.e., four grams of alcohol diluted to 40 percent.]

If the patient is exceptionally excitable and sensitive, one takes a teaspoon or coffee spoon of the solution from this glass, after stirring it vigorously, and again very vigorously stirs it into a second drinking glass of water and gives the patient a coffee spoon, or a little more, of this.

There are patients who are so sensitive that one has to dilute the solution in a third or fourth drinking glass in this manner for them.

Each day after each dose of the remedy, one throws out what is left in the glass or glasses; each glass of solution is made fresh every time it is used.

It is best to crush the globule of highly potentized medicine into a few grains* of powdered milk sugar so that all the patient has to do is put it into the bottle that holds the correct amount of water.

249

Any medicine that during its action brings about new and perhaps troublesome symptoms not characteristic of the case cannot effect a real improvement and should not be considered to have been chosen homoeopathically.[a] If the aggravation is serious, it must be somewhat reduced by an antidote as soon as possible[b] before one gives the next remedy more accurately chosen for the similarity of its action. But if the adverse symptoms are not too violent, the correctly chosen remedy must be given immediately to replace the incorrectly chosen one. .

a. Since according to all experience almost no dose of a highly potentized, specifically appropriate homoeopathic medicine can be too small to bring about a clear improvement in the disease for which it is suited (par. 161, par. 279), one would be treating wrongly

*[See translators' note to par. 270.]

and harmfully if, as happens in the old school, one were to repeat or indeed even increase the dose of that medicine when there was no improvement or when there was slight aggravation, in the mistaken belief that the medicine was not able to help because the amount (the size of the dose) was too small. *Any aggravation involving new symptoms*—if there has been no error in the patient's mental or physical regimen—*always means only that the previous remedy was inappropriate* to the case: *it never means that the dose was too weak.*

b. There can never be any case in the practice of a well-trained, scrupulously careful physician in which he would have to give an antidote, if he starts—as he should do—with the smallest possible dose of his well-chosen medicine, because an equally small dose of a better-chosen medicine would correct any mistake he might make.

250

Thus, in an urgent case, when an observant physician who pays careful attention to his patient's condition notices after six, eight, or twelve hours that his last remedy was incorrectly chosen, because the patient is unmistakably worse by the hour, no matter how slightly, and that new symptoms and complaints are arising, he is not only allowed to rectify his mistake but duty bound to do so; he must find and administer a homoeopathic remedy that is not just fairly well indicated for the disease condition as it now is but is as well indicated as possible (par. 167).

251

There are a few medicines, such as *Ignatia, Bryonia,* and *Rhus toxicodendron,* and, to a degree, *Belladonna,* whose abilities to change human health consist mainly of alternating actions—primary-action symptoms somewhat opposite to each other. If after prescribing one of these on strictly homoeopathic principles the physician finds that there is no improvement, he will in most cases quickly achieve his objective (in acute diseases after a few hours) by giving a second, equally small dose of the same medicine.[a]

a. As I have explained in detail in the introduction to *Ignatia* in my *Materia Medica Pura*.

252

But if, apart from these, one finds in a chronic case that the best chosen homoeopathic medicine given in the correct (smallest) dose does not bring about improvement, then it is a *certain* sign that an influence sustaining the disease still persists and that there is something in the patient's way of life or environment which must be eliminated if permanent cure is to be achieved.

253

In all diseases, especially in quickly arising (acute) ones, of all the signs that indicate a small beginning of improvement or aggravation that is not visible to everybody, the psychic condition of the patient and his general demeanor are the most certain and revealing. The very beginning of improvement is indicated by a sense of greater ease, composure, mental freedom, higher spirits, and returning naturalness. The very beginning of aggravation, on the other hand, is indicated by the opposite—a more constrained, helpless, pitiable state with regard to his emotions, mind, general demeanor, attitude, posture, and actions, which can easily be seen and pointed out if one is attentive but cannot be described in words.[a]

a. The signs of improvement in the emotions and mind can be expected immediately after the medicine has been taken only if the dose was *small enough* (i.e., as small as possible); an unnecessarily larger dose even of the most homoeopathically appropriate remedy, apart from its other ill effects (par. 276), acts too violently and initially disturbs the mind and emotions too strongly and too long for the patient's improvement to be noticed *immediately*.

Here I would like to say that brash beginners in homoeopathy and converts from the old school are the ones who most frequently transgress this essential rule. Out of inveterate prejudice they are reluctant to use the smallest doses of the higher dynamizations and must therefore sacrifice the great advantages and blessings of this procedure, which experience has shown thousands of times to be the most curative; they do not achieve that which genuine homoeopathy can do and thus wrongly claim to be its disciples.

254

For the observant and penetrating physician, either the appearance of other symptoms that are new and foreign to the disease being treated or else the decline of the original symptoms without any new ones will soon dispel any doubt that may remain about the aggravation or improvement, even in those patients who are either unable to tell or unwilling to admit that their general condition is better or worse.

255

Even with such patients, one will be able to reach a conclusion by going through the records of their cases with them and reviewing the symptoms one by one. If one finds in addition to mental and emotional improvement already observed that they cannot complain of any new, unfamiliar symptoms, while none of the old ones are worse, then the medicine must have brought about an essential reduction of the disease or, if there has not been enough time, will soon do so. If obvious improvement does not ensue promptly, the fault lies in the patient's behavior or in some other circumstances impeding the improvement.

256

On the other hand, if the patient complains of some significant new symptoms, symptoms belonging to the remedy that was not homoeopathically correct, even if he good-naturedly assures us that he is feeling better,[a] we should not heed this assurance, but consider his condition to be worse, which will soon be clearly evident.

a. This is not rare among consumptives with pulmonary suppuration.

257

The true physician will be careful to avoid making favorites of certain remedies that he has happened to have found indicated rather often and has had the opportunity of employing with good results. Otherwise, less frequently used remedies that might be more homoeopathically suitable and therefore more helpful will often be overlooked.

258

Conversely, in treating new cases, the true physician will not be oversuspicious and disregard remedies that he has now and then used with bad results through improper selection (and therefore by his own fault). He will not avoid these remedies for any reason other than that they are unhomoeopathic to the case, mindful that the only medicinal disease agent meriting attention and preference in any case of disease is always the one that is most similar to the totality of the characteristic symptoms and that no petty bias should interfere with this serious choice.

259

Considering the smallness of the dose, which in homoeopathy is as necessary as it is effective, it is easy to understand that during treatment everything that could have any medicinal action must be removed from the *diet* and the daily *regimen,* so that the subtle dose is not overwhelmed and extinguished, not even disturbed, by any foreign medicinal influence.[a]

a. The soft, distant sounds of the flute in the silence of midnight, which would lift the tender heart to divine ecstacy and melt it in religious fervor, are drowned out to ineffectiveness in the noisy din of day, which is foreign to them.

260

For the chronically ill it is all the more necessary to seek out carefully such obstacles to cure, because the disease has usually been aggravated by such harmful medicinal influences and by other errors of living which often go unrecognized.[a]

a. Coffee, fine China tea, and other herbal teas; beers adulterated with medicinal vegetable substances unsuitable to the patient's condition; so-called fine liqueurs made from medicinal spices; all kinds of cordials; spiced chocolate; toilet waters and all kinds of perfumes; strong-smelling flowers in the room; medicinal dentifrices; perfumed sachets; highly spiced food and sauces; spiced pastry and ice cream prepared with such medicinal substances as coffee and vanilla; crude medicinal herbs in soups; vegetable dishes of herbs, roots, and sprouts (such as asparagus with long green tips); hops sprouts and all medicinal vegetables, including celery, parsley, sorrel, tarragon, all kinds of onions, etc.; old cheese and meat that is not fresh or that has medicinal effects (the flesh or fat of pork, ducks, and geese, veal that is too young, pickled meats, and all kinds of hors d'oeuvres): all these things should be kept from such patients.

They should in the same way avoid any excess in such things as sugar and salt; undiluted alcoholic drinks; room heating; woolen underwear; sedentary living in enclosed quarters; frequent merely passive movement (riding, driving, swinging); excessive nursing; prolonged siestas; reading while lying down; keeping late hours; uncleanliness; unnatural debauchery; enervation from salacious reading; onanism or, in marriage, coitus interruptus or complete abstinence—either from superstition or to prevent conception; an environment in which there is anger, grief, vexation; overindulgence in games; overexertion of mind and body, especially after meals; marshy habitation and damp rooms; penury; etc. All these things must be eliminated or else avoided as much as possible if cure is not to be prevented or impeded. Some of my imitators unnecessarily make the patient's regimen even harder and forbid many more rather unimportant things, which is not to be condoned.

261

In chronic diseases the best way of living while taking medicine is achieved by the elimination of these impediments to recovery and, whenever called for, the inclusion of their opposites: innocent recreations of mind and emotions, outdoor exercise in almost any kind of weather (daily walks, light manual labor), suitable, nourishing, nonmedicinal food and drink, etc.

262

In acute diseases, on the other hand—except if the patient is delirious—the subtle, dependable, inner life-preserving instinct (here very active) speaks so clearly and unmistakably that the physician needs only to instruct the family and attendants not to thwart this voice of nature by denying the patient food he craves or pressing on him what he does not want.

263

Of course, the acutely ill patient desires for the most part only foods and drinks that bring him palliative relief, which fulfill only the needs of the moment and are not actually medicines. If the gratification of these desires *remains within the limits of moderation,* the slight obstacles that they might perhaps place in the way of real cure[a] will be amply overcome and outweighed by the strength of the appropriate homoeopathic medicine and the vital principle, which it has set free, and by the comfort that the patient has derived from the satisfaction of his craving. In acute diseases the warmth of the room and of the bed must likewise be entirely to the patient's desire. He should be kept from all mental exertion and emotional disturbance.

a. These are, however, rare. Thus, for example, in purely inflammatory disease where *Aconite* is indispensable but would be neutralized by vegetable acid, the patient almost always craves only pure cold water.

264

The true physician must have available *authentic medicines in perfect condition* if he is to depend on their therapeutic power. He must know *for himself* that they are genuine.

265

It is for him a matter of conscience to be absolutely sure that the patient always receives the right medicine. Therefore he *himself* must provide the patient with the correctly chosen remedy, which he *himself* has prepared.[a]

a. To uphold this very important basic principle of my teaching I have endured much persecution since discovering it.

266

Substances from the animal and vegetable kingdoms are most medicinally active in their crude state.[a]

a. All crude animal and vegetable substances have more or less medicinal virtue and can alter the state of human health, each in its own way.

Plants and animals that the most enlightened nations use for food have the merit of being more nutritious and differ from the others in that the medicinal qualities of their crude state, already not very strong, are reduced by cooking and domestic preparation: by pressing out the harmful juice (as with the cassava root in South America); by fementation—of flour in dough in making bread, in sauerkraut made without vinegar, in brine-cured cucumbers; by smoking; by the action of heat (in boiling, stewing, roasting, grilling, or baking, and for potatoes, thorough steaming).

By these means the medicinal part of many such substances is to a degree destroyed and dissipated. Animal and vegetable substances do lose much of their medicinal harmfulness through the addition of salt (in pickling) and vinegar (in sauces and salads) but acquire other disadvantages from these additions.

Even the most medicinally potent plants partly or even entirely lose their power through such treatment. By complete desiccation the roots of iris, horseradish, arum, and peony lose almost all their medicinal power. The sap of the most poisonous plants often becomes a totally inert, tarry mass from the heat involved in the preparation of ordinary extracts. The expressed sap of the most deadly plants becomes entirely inert just from the long exposure to the air; at moderate air temperature it soon ferments spontaneously, like wine, and thereby loses much of its medicinal power, and immediately after that it proceeds through a stage like vinegar fermentation and then putrefies and loses all its medicinal characteristics; if the starchy sediment deposited is washed, it is completely innocuous like any other starch; even the sweating that takes place when green herbs are piled up on top of each other removes most of their medicinal power.

267

To utilize in the most complete and certain way the power of indigenous plants that can be obtained fresh, one thoroughly mixes the sap, *immediately* after it has been pressed out, with an equal amount of wine spirit strong enough for a sponge to burn in it. One then lets this stand for twenty-four hours in a tightly closed bottle, and decants the clear liquid from the fibrous and albuminous matter that has settled, and stores it carefully for medicinal use.[a] The wine spirit immediately stops all fermentation of the sap and makes subsequent fermentation impossible. By this method the medicinal strength of the sap can be *permanently* preserved perfect and unspoiled, stored away from the sunlight in bottles that have been well closed and sealed with molten wax to prevent evaporation.[b]

a. Bucholz (*Taschenb. f. Scheidek. u. Apoth. a. d. J.*, Weimar, 1815, vols. I, VI) assures his readers (and his reviewer in the *Leipziger Literaturzeitung,* 1816, No. 82, did not contradict him) that we owe this superlative method of preparing medicines to the Russian campaign of 1812 whence it reached Germany in 1813. Following the noble custom of many Germans to deny the merits of their compatriots, he conceals the fact that this discovery and these directions, which he quotes *in my own words* from the first edition of the *Organon of Rational Medicine* (par. 230 and note), came from me and that I gave them to the world *for the first time* in that book two years before the Russian campaign (the *Organon* appeared in 1810). These people would rather pretend that a discovery came from the wilds of Asia than give a German just credit for it. Oh, the manners and ways of our time!

Of course, before this, one sometimes mixed the sap of plants with wine spirit to store it for a while before making an extract from it, but never with the intention of administering it in this form.

b. Equal parts of wine spirit and freshly pressed sap usually make up the right proportion for precipitating the fibrous and albuminous matter.

For plants that contain much mucilage (e.g., *Symphytum officinale* roots and *Viola tricolor,* etc.) or an excess of albumin (e.g., *Aethusa cynapium, Solanum nigrum,* etc.) one usually needs a double proportion of alcohol.

Very dry plants, such as *Oleander, Buxus, Taxus, Ledum, Sabina,* etc., must first be powdered alone into a fine moist pulp and then stirred into a double portion of wine spirit, with which the sap combines so that, thus extracted, it can be pressed out. One can also bring them to the one-millionth trituration in sugar of milk after drying (if one uses sufficient force during the trituration) and then, after dissolving a grain of this,* one can make further liquid dynamizations (par. 271).

268

Exotic plants, barks, seeds, and roots, which cannot be obtained fresh, will never be accepted in powdered form by the sensible physician on trust; he will make sure that they are genuine while they are still in crude, unpowdered form and before making any medicinal use of them whatsoever.[a]

*[See translators' footnote, par. 270.]

a. In order to preserve them in powdered form, one has to take a precaution that was previously almost unknown to pharmacists, so that they could not even preserve powders of well-dried animal and vegetable substances in well-closed bottles without spoilage.

Even fully dried whole, crude vegetable substances necessarily contain a certain amount of moisture to hold their fabric together; this is not enough to allow the drug to spoil when it is whole and unpowdered but quite enough when it is finely powdered. Thus animal and vegetable substances that have been completely dried while still whole produce on pulverization a somewhat moist powder that cannot be stored in tightly closed bottles without rapidly molding and decaying unless this excess of moisture has first been removed.

The best way to do this is to spread the powder in a flat, high-sided tin dish floating in a pot of boiling water (i.e., in a water bath) and dry it by stirring until its particles no longer stick together but easily separate and scatter like fine dry sand. In this dry state the fine powder can be *permanently* stored at its original medicinal strength in a well-closed and sealed bottle without spoiling and *without ever becoming mite ridden or moldy*. Preferably it should be protected from light in a closed canister, box, or container. All animal and vegetable substances gradually lose their medicinal strength even when they are whole, and far more when they are powdered, if they are not stored in airtight containers away from light.

269

For its own special purpose and by its own special procedure, never tried before my time, homoeopathy develops the inner, spirit-like medicinal powers of crude substance to a degree hitherto unheard of and makes all of them exceedingly, even immeasurably, penetrating, active, and effective, *even those that in the crude state do not have the slightest medicinal effect on the human organism.*[a]

This remarkable transformation of the properties of natural bodies through the mechanical action of trituration and succussion on their tiniest particles (*while these particles are diffused in an inert dry or liquid substance*) develops the latent *dynamic* (par. 11) powers previously imperceptible and as it were lying hidden asleep in them.[b] These powers electively affect the vital principle of animal life.[c] This process is called *dynamization* or *potentization* (development of medicinal power), and it creates what we call *dynamizations* or *potencies* of different degrees.[d]

a. Long before I made this discovery, people were aware through experience of different changes that can be produced in various natural substances *by friction*—for instance, warmth, heat, fire; the development of odor in odorless objects; the magnetization of steel; etc. But all these properties produced by friction manifested only on a lifeless, physical level, whereas there is a law of nature by which physiological and pathogenetic forces capable of altering the health of living organisms are generated in the crude substance of a remedy through trituration and succussion, even a substance never before found to be medicinal, provided it is diffused in fixed proportions of an inert, nonmedicinal medium. This wonderful law, which is physical but more especially physiological and pathogenetic, was not known before me.

It is no wonder, then, that natural scientists and

physicians of our day (*still unfamiliar with this*) have not hitherto believed in the magical healing powers of remedies prepared according to the homoeopathic method (dynamized) and employed in such small doses!

b. In the same way there is no denying that there is within an iron bar or a steel rod a slumbering trace of magnetic force. When either has been left standing upright immediately after being forged, its lower end repels the north pole of a magnetic needle and attracts the south pole, while in the same way the upper end proves to be a south pole. But this is only a *latent* force; not even the finest iron filings can be magnetically attracted or held by either end of such a rod. Not until we have *dynamized* a steel rod, rubbing it *strongly in one direction* with a blunt file, does it become a true, active, powerful magnet capable of attracting iron and steel and of imparting magnetism to another steel rod not just by contact but even at some distance; the more it has been rubbed, the more strongly this happens.

Similarly, by the trituration of a medicinal substance and the succussion of its solution (*dynamization, potentization*) the medicinal forces lying hidden in it are developed and uncovered more and more, and the material is itself spiritualized, if one may use that expression.

c. Therefore, this transformation is the increase and greater development only of the power that these natural bodies have to affect humans and animals in their *state of health* when, in their refined condition, they touch or closely approach sensitive living tissue (through ingestion or inhalation); just as a magnet (more so if its magnetism has been increased, dynamized) will produce in a steel needle near or touching its pole only magnetism, without changing the steel in any of its other physical or chemical properties. And just as the magnet will not bring about any change in other metals, such as brass, so also dynamized medicines do not affect lifeless things.

d. Every day one still hears homoeopathic medicinal potencies referred to as *mere dilutions,* while they are in fact quite the opposite: trituration and succussion unlock the natural substances, uncover and reveal the specific medicinal powers lying hidden in their soul. The nonmedicinal dilutant is only an *auxiliary, though indispensable, factor.*

Simple dilution, e.g., of a grain of salt, results in nothing but pure water. The grain of salt disappears upon being diluted in a large amount of water and never thereby becomes the medicinal salt that our properly made dynamizations have raised to such a wonderful power.

270

[Translators' note: Hahnemann speaks of a grain. The standard Troy grain of the time corresponds to exactly 0.064798918 grams in our metric system. But according to the second edition of the German *Pharmacopoeia,* 1950, Hahnemann used the Nuremberg measure: one grain was 0.062 grams in our system. If Hahnemann had lived today it is almost certain that he would have indicated 0.05 grams as a practical quantity easy to work with.

Hahnemann speaks of *Branntwein,* which we have translated as "brandywine": this is equivalent to our 90 degree grain alcohol. When he speaks of *guter Weingeist,* which we have translated as "rectified wine spirit," this is equivalent to our 95 degree grain alcohol.]

Now, to develop this power most effectively, a small quantity of the substance to be dynamized, about a grain, is raised to the one-millionth attenuation in powder [third centesimal trituration, or 3 C] by making three hour-long triturations with 100 grains of milk sugar each time, as explained below.[a] For reasons explained in footnote *f,* a grain of this triturate is first of all dissolved in 500 drops of a mixture of one part brandywine and four parts distilled water, and a *single drop* of this is put in a vial. One adds 100 drops of rectified wine spirit[b] to this and gives 100 strong succussions to the tightly closed vial by hand against a hard but elastic object.[c] This is the medicine in the *first* degree of dynamization. One thoroughly moistens[d] tiny sugar globules[e] with this, then rapidly spreads them out on filter paper, dries them, and stores them in a tightly closed bottle labeled I, the first degree of potency. From this, a single globule[f] is taken for further dynamization and put (with 1 drop of water to dissolve it) into another, second vial, then dynamized in 100 drops of rectified wine spirit by means of 100 strong succussions, as before. Once again globules are moistened with this medicinal spirit, rapidly spread out on filter paper, dried, stored in a tightly closed bottle protected from heat and light, and labeled II, the second degree of potency. One proceeds in this way until a dissolved globule of XXIX (the twenty-ninth degree of potency) is succussed with 100 drops of rectified wine spirit by means of 100 strong succussions to form a medicinal spirit, and globules moistened with this and dried are labeled XXX, the thirtieth degree of dynamization.

Only after crude medicinal substances have been processed in this way does one obtain preparations that have attained their full power to affect the suffering parts of the sick organism with a similar artificial disease so as to remove from the indwelling vital principle its sensation of the natural disease. If this mechanical process is properly carried out according to these instructions, the medicinal substance that seems to us in its crude state only matter, sometimes even nonmedicinal matter, is at last completely transformed and refined by these progressive dynamizations to become a spirit-like medicinal force.[g] This spirit-like medicinal force *by itself* is no longer perceptible to the senses, but the medicated globule acts as its *carrier* and demonstrates its curative power in the sick organism even when used dry, but far more when dissolved in water.

a. One puts one-third of 100 grains of powdered milk sugar in a glazed porcelain mortar, the bottom of which one has roughened by rubbing with fine, moist sand, and adds *on top* of this powder 1 grain of the pulverized medicinal substance to be prepared (1 drop of mercury, petroleum, etc.). The milk sugar that is to be used for dynamization must be of the special, pure quality that comes in round sticks crystallized on threads. One mixes the medicine and the powder together with a porcelain spatula for a moment and triturates the mixture rather strongly for six or seven minutes with a porcelain pestle that has also been roughened at the bottom, then for about three or four minutes thoroughly scrapes the mass from the bottom of the mortar and the pestle to make it homogeneous; again for six or seven minutes one triturates with the same force, without adding anything, and then scrapes the triturate from the bottom of both mortar and pestle for three or four minutes. At this point one adds the second third of the milk sugar, stirs everything together with a spatula for a moment, and then triturates it for six or seven minutes with the same force and again scrapes it for three or four minutes; again one continues the trituration for six or seven minutes without adding anything and scrapes for three or four minutes. At this point one adds the last third of the milk sugar, stirs with the spatula, strongly triturates again for six or seven minutes, scrapes it all together for three or four minutes, and finally finishes by triturating for the last six or seven minutes and scraping very carefully.

The powder prepared in this way is stored in a tightly closed vial protected from light and labeled with the name of the substance and the number 1/100 [one-hundredth attenuation, or first centesimal trituration, 1 C].

Now in order to raise this product to the one ten-thousandth attenuation [second centesimal trituration, or 2 C], one puts one grain of this powder of the first centesimal attenuation into the mortar with a third of 100 grains of powdered milk sugar, mixes everything together with the spatula, and proceeds as above. One must make sure that each third is strongly triturated twice before the next third is added, and each time for about six or seven minutes, followed by three or four minutes of scraping. For each third one proceeds exactly as before. When this is done one puts the powder in a tightly closed vial and labels it 1/10,000.

If one again continues in this way with one grain of this last powder, one raises it to the one one-millionth attentuation [third centesimal trituration, or 3 C] so that each grain of this powder contains one-millionth of a grain of the original substance.

Each of the three degrees of such a powder preparation requires six times six or seven minutes of trituration and six times three or four minutes of scraping, making a total of *one hour.*

After the first hour-long trituration each grain of the preparation contains one one-hundreth grain of the substance being used; after the second hour-long trituration it contains one ten-thousandth grain of the substance; after the third and final hour-long trituration it contains one one-millionth grain of the substance.*

The mortar, pestle, and spatula must be thoroughly cleaned before being used to prepare another medicine. They are to be well washed in hot water and carefully dried, then thoroughly boiled for a half hour in a kettle of water; one might then even take the precaution of setting these utensils on top of coals that are just starting to glow.

b. The potentizing vial is filled to two-thirds with this liquid.

c. E.g., a leather-bound book.

d. One puts the globules to be medicated into a small thimble-shaped vessel made of glass, porcelain, or silver, with a small opening in the bottom: one moistens them with some of the medicinally dynamized wine spirit, stirs them, and then inverts the little vessel over a sheet of filter paper and taps out the tiny globules onto it to dry them quickly.

e. These should be made out of starch flour and cane sugar by a confectioner under one's own supervision. The fine dustlike particles are first of all sifted from these tiny globules; then they are put through a sieve with holes through which *only those weighing 1 grain per 100* can pass. This is the most useful size for the requirements of the homoeopathic physician.

f. According to my earlier instructions a whole drop of the liquid in the lower potency always had to be added to 100 drops of wine spirit for further potentization. But meticulous experiments have convinced me that this ratio between the quantity of the dilutant and that of the medicine being dynamized (100:1) is far too low to develop the medicinal sub-

---

*These are the three degrees of dry powder trituration, which, when well executed, have already made a good beginning toward developing the power of the medicinal substance (dynamization).

stance properly and to a high degree with a large number of succussions unless force is used. Whereas if one takes a single globule, 100 of which weigh a grain, and dynamizes it with 100 drops of wine spirit, then the ratio becomes 50,000:1, indeed higher than that, because 500 of such globules cannot completely absorb 1 drop. In this much higher ratio between dilutant and medicinal substance *a large number* of succussions of the vial filled to two-thirds with wine spirit can bring about a far greater development of power.

When the ratio of dilutant to medicine is as low as 100:1 if very many succussions are, as it were, forced into it by a powerful machine, we obtain medicines that, especially in the higher degrees of dynamization, act almost instantaneously but with intense, even dangerous violence, particularly on delicate patients, without bringing about the permanent, gentle counteraction of the vital principle.

But my new method produces medicines of the highest power and the mildest action which, if well chosen, heal all the sick parts of the organism.*

Using these far more perfectly dynamized medicines, one can in acute fevers repeat the small doses of the lowest degrees of dynamization even at short intervals and even with medicines of long action, such as *Belladonna*. And in chronic diseases one can best proceed by beginning the treatment with the lowest degrees of dynamization and if necessary continue to the higher degrees, which are increasingly strong but always act gently.

---

*Only in the very rare cases where a troublesome inveterate local affection persists though health is already almost completely restored and the vital force is strong is it permitted, even *absolutely necessary*, to administer progressively larger doses of the medicine found to be homoeopathically beneficial, but only after it has been potentized to a very high degree by succussing it many times by hand. Such a local affection then often miraculously disappears very quickly.

g. This assertion will not appear implausible if one considers that with this method of dynamization (whose products I have found after many painstaking experiments and counterexperiments to be the strongest and at the same time the mildest, i.e., the most perfect) the material quantity of the medicine is reduced 50,000 times with each degree of dynamization, and yet its power increases incredibly. If we multiply by the base number of 50,000 at each progressive dynamization, the material substance is already reduced 125×10^{18} times at the third potency [the one one-millionth of the original third centesimal trituration multiplied by $50,000^3$]. It therefore follows that the thirtieth degree of dynamization represents a fraction that could hardly be written out any more.

It is highly probable that during such dynamization (development of its true, inner medicinal nature) the material substance eventually dissolves completely into its individual spirit-like essence and that its crude state can be regarded as actually consisting only of this spirit-like essence, as yet undeveloped.

271

If the physician prepares his homoeopathic medicines himself, which is what he should do if he is to liberate mankind from diseases,[a] he can use fresh plants themselves, since only a small amount of crude substance is required—unless he happens to need the extracted juice for purposes of treatment. He will put a few grains of the fresh plant in the mortar and bring it to the one one-millionth attenuation [third centesimal trituration] (par. 270), with three times 100 grains of milk sugar, and then proceed to further potentization by dissolving a small part of this triturate and succussing it. One also proceeds in this manner with all other crude medicinal substances of a dry or oily nature.

a. Until such time as the state, realizing the necessity of perfectly prepared homoeopathic medicines, has them prepared by a capable, disinterested individual so that they may be given without charge to homoeopathic physicians of the country who have been instructed in healing in homoeopathic hospitals, tested in theory and practice, and thus certified. In this way not only will the physician be assured of the quality of these divine instruments of healing, but he will be able to give them free to patients rich and poor.

272

One such globule placed dry on the tongue is one of the smallest doses for a mild disease of recent onset.[a] Here only a few nerve endings are touched by the medicine. But an identical globule crushed into some milk sugar and dissolved into a large amount of water (par. 247) and well shaken before each dose provides a far stronger medicine for use over several days. Each dose of it, however small, immediately touches many nerve endings.

a. These globules (see par. 270) retain their medicinal power for *many* years if protected from sunlight and heat.

273

In no case being treated is it necessary to give a patient more than a *single simple* medicinal substance at one time, and *for this reason by itself it is inadmissible to do so.* It is inconceivable that there could be the slightest doubt about whether it is more natural and rational to prescribe a *single simple,*[a] well-known medicinal substance or a mixture of many different ones for a patient at any one time. In homoeopathy, the only true and simple natural therapy, it is absolutely forbidden to give the patient two different medicinal substances *at any one time.*

a. Neutral and intermediate salts formed through chemical affinity from two opposite substances in fixed proportions; naturally occurring sulphuretted metals and compounds of sulphur with alkaline salts and earths formed artificially in fixed proportions (e.g., sodium or calcium compounds of sulphur); ethers formed by combining alcohol and acids through distillation; and phosphorus: these can be accepted by homoeopathic physicians as *simple* medicinal substances and used to treat patients.

On the other hand, so-called alkaloids extracted from plants by using acids (e.g., quinine, strychnine, morphine) are subject to great variations in their preparation and therefore cannot be accepted by the homoeopathic physician as simple, unvarying medicines, especially since he already has in the plants themselves in their natural condition (cinchona bark, Nux vomica, opium) all that he needs from them for curing. Besides, alkaloids are not the only medicinal constituents of plants.

274

The true physician already finds in simple medicines employed unmixed and by themselves everything he could wish for—artificial disease agents that can by their homoeopathic power completely overcome natural diseases, extinguish them in the feelings of the vital principle, permanently cure them. So it will never occur to him to administer more than one simple medicinal substance at a time—in accordance with the wise saying that it is wrong to use complex means when simple ones will do. Because even if each medicine has been *fully proved* by itself to determine its pure characteristic effects on the healthy, if two or more of them are given together it is still impossible to predict just *how* they might interfere with each other and alter each other in their effects on the human organism. And because in cases where the symptom totality is precisely known, a simple medicinal substance by itself already cures completely if it is homoeopathic.

Even in the worst of cases, where the remedy could not be chosen in exact accordance with the symptom totality and where it therefore has not cured, the new complaints that the remedy produces nevertheless serve to further our knowledge of medicines by confirming the symptoms that this substance has produced on the healthy human organism, an advantage of which we are deprived when more than one medicine is used at the same time.[a]

a. After the rational physician has carefully considered a case and given internally the right homoeopathic remedy, to have the patient drink infusions of other medicinal substances, apply a poultice or fomentation of different herbs, take a dissimilar clyster, or rub in some salve or other is something that he leaves to the irrational routine of the allopaths.

275

The correctness of a medicine for a given case of disease depends not only on its accurate homoeopathic selection but also on the correct size (or rather small-ness) of the dose. A medicine given in *too large a dose,* though completely homoeopathic to the case and in it-self of a beneficial nature, will still harm the patient by its quantity and unnecessarily strong action on the vital force, and through it, because the medicine is homoeo-pathic, on precisely those parts of the organism which are most sensitive and have already been afflicted most by the natural disease.

276

For this reason a medicine, although homoeopathic to the case, does harm when it is given in overdose. In strong doses the more homoeopathic the medicine and the higher its potency the more harm it does:[a] indeed it is far more harmful than equally large doses of unho-moeopathic medicine, an allopathic one unrelated to the disease condition. Excessively large doses of an accu-rately selected homoeopathic medicine, especially if fre-quently repeated, are, as a rule, very destructive. Not infrequently, they endanger the patient's life or make his disease almost incurable. Of course they do extin-guish the natural disease in the feelings of the vital prin-ciple—the patient no longer suffers from it as soon as the overdose of homoeopathic medicine acts on him; but he is then more seriously ill from the completely similar but far stronger medicinal disease, which is ex-tremely difficult to eradicate.[b]

a. The great praise that some homoeopathic physi-cians have recently lavished upon larger doses stems in part from the fact that they use lower potencies dynamized according to my earlier method (more or less as I myself did many years ago for want of better knowledge), partly from the fact that their medicines were not chosen homoeopathically, and partly because the manufacturer had prepared them very imperfectly.

b. In this way almost incurable mercury cachexias arise from continued large, violent, allopathically prescribed doses of mercurial remedies for syphilis, when one or a few doses of a mild but effective mercurial remedy would no doubt have cured the entire venereal disease completely within a few days, including the chancre, if this had not been suppressed by external remedies (which is what allopathy always does).

The allopath likewise gives large doses of cinchona bark and quinine day after day for intermittent fevers, often when they are indeed homoeopathically indicated, and a very small dose of *highly* potentized *China* would certainly have helped (in marsh fever where the patient is indeed not suffering from manifest psora). He thereby produces a chronic quinine cachexia (and awakens the psora), which, if it does not gradually kill the patient, at least causes him to suffer a dismal state of health for years by destroying his vital organs, especially the liver and spleen. A homoeopathic antidote for such a condition caused by the excessive use of large doses of a homoeopathic medicine is hardly conceivable.

277

For the same reason and since, if the dose is appropriately small, a well-dynamized medicine becomes increasingly curative and almost miraculously helpful the more homoeopathically it has been chosen, it follows that if a medicine is accurately homoeopathic it must become increasingly beneficial as its dose approaches the ideal degree of smallness for gentle action.

278

Now the question arises what this ideal degree of smallness is, the degree that is certain and gentle in its remedial effect: how small should the dose of a given correctly chosen homoeopathic medicine be to cure a case of disease in the best way? To solve this problem, to determine for a given medicine used in homoeopathic practice what dose would be sufficient and at the same time small enough to effect the gentlest, quickest cure, is not a matter of theoretical conjecture, as one can easily understand. Theorizing and specious sophistry cannot enlighten us on this subject, nor can every possible eventuality be tabulated in advance. Only pure experiment, the meticulous observation of the sensitivity of each patient, and sound experience can determine this *in each individual case.*

It would be foolish to disregard what pure experience teaches us about the smallness of the dose necessary for homoeopathic cure and to favor the large doses of the inappropriate (allopathic) medicines of the old school, which do not homoeopathically affect the sick part of the organism, but only attack the part that the disease has not taken hold of.

279

Pure experience *absolutely* proves that even in a chronic or complicated disease, when there is no extensive damage to some vital organ, and though all other foreign medicinal influence has been withheld from the patient, *the dose of the highly potentized homoeopathic remedy beginning the treatment of a significant (chronic) disease can, as a rule, not be made so small*

that it is not stronger than the natural disease,
that it cannot at least partially overcome it,

*that it cannot at least partially extinguish it in the
    feelings of the vital principle,
that it cannot start the process of cure.*

280

One continues to give a medicine as long as it continues to benefit the patient and does not give rise to any new troublesome complaints, and one *gradually increases the dose* until the patient, *while feeling generally better,* begins once again to experience one or more of his old, original symptoms to a moderate degree. If the remedy has been modified each time by succussion (par. 247) and the very moderate doses have been gradually increased, this return of old symptoms indicates that cure is imminent, and that the vital principle has almost no more need to be affected by the similar medicinal disease in order to stop feeling the natural disease (par. 148), and that, now more free of the natural disease, it is beginning to suffer somewhat from the homoeopathic medicinal disease, otherwise known as *homoeopathic aggravation.*

281

To confirm this, one leaves the patient without medicine for a week or two and gives him only some powdered milk sugar during this time. If the last few symptoms come only from the medicine's mimicking the previous ones, they will go away within a few days or hours, and, provided the patient continues to live properly, no more traces of the original disease will manifest themselves during the period without medicine, meaning that the patient will in all probability have been cured.

But if, on the other hand, traces of the previous disease symptoms are still manifesting at the end of this period without medicine, they are remains of the original disease, which has not yet been completely extinguished: treatment must be resumed with higher degrees of dynamization, in the manner taught above.

The first, smallest doses must, of course, as before, be increased gradually in order to cure. But for patients in whom one observes considerable sensitivity, the doses are increased far more slowly, and by far smaller amounts than for patients who are less sensitive, for whom the doses can be more rapidly increased. There are patients who are unusually sensitive, a thousand times more sensitive than those who are least sensitive.

282

If during treatment, especially of a chronic disease, the first doses already produce a so-called *homoeopathic aggravation,* i.e., a noticeable heightening of the disease symptoms originally observed, even though each repeated dose was somewhat modified (more highly dynamized) by succussion (par. 247), then this is a sure sign that the doses were too large.[a]

a. There is a very important exception to the rule that the homoeopathic treatment of chronic diseases must begin with the smallest possible doses and that these doses must be increased only very gradually: when the three great miasms are still manifesting on the skin (newly arisen *scabies,* undisturbed syphilitic *chancres* on the genitals, the labia, the lips, etc. and *fig-warts*) they not only can but actually must be treated at the very beginning with large doses of their specific remedy given in increasing degrees of dynamization once, even perhaps several times a day. In such cases one need have no fear that an excessively large dose, though extinguishing the disease, could cause a medicinal disease and if repeated, a chronic one. This is what happens when a disease concealed inside the organism is treated in this way, but it does not happen when the primary manifestations of these three miasms are openly visible, since one can actually see in their day by day improvement how much the daily large dose has removed the disease from the feelings of the vital principle. None of these three miasms can be cured without indicating to the physician by the disappearance of their primary symptoms that no more medicine is necessary.

Since all diseases are only dynamic disturbances of the vital principle and are not caused by anything material, by any *materia peccans* (a fiction that the old school in its delusion has preached and by which it has treated for thousands of years, always to the ruin of its patients), there is nothing material in these cases either, nothing that can be removed, rubbed or burned away, tied or cut off, without making the patient, for the rest of his life, infinitely more sick and incurable than he ever was with the undisturbed primary manifestations of these three great miasms (see *Chronic Diseases,* vol. I).

These external signs of the internal, virulent miasms are caused by a dynamic influence inimical to the vital principle; they can be extinguished only by a homoeopathic medicine acting on the vital principle in a similar manner but more strongly. The homoeopathic medicine removes from the vital principle its sensation of the inner and outer spirit-like disease agent, which then no longer exists for it (for the organism), so that the patient is left cured and free of disease.

Experience shows that scabies, along with its eruption, and syphilis, along with its chancre, can and must be cured only with the specific medicine internally administered; fig-warts, however, when they have remained untreated for some time, require for complete cure that their specific medicine be applied externally at the same time as it is used internally.

283

To do things in the most natural way—and even for this reason alone—the true physician prescribes his medicines, which he has in all respects chosen in the most homoeopathic way, in the smallest possible doses. And because these doses are so small, if through human weakness he chooses a medicine rather inappropriate to the disease, the harm done would be so insignificant that it would quickly be overcome and corrected by the life-force itself and by the counterinfluence of a more similar remedy immediately administered (par. 249) in the same minute dose.

284

In addition to the tongue, the mouth,[a] and the stomach, the places through which medicine most usually affects the organism, the nose and respiratory organs are especially sensitive to medicines in liquid form if they are smelled or if their vapors are inhaled through the mouth. The skin and epidermis of the whole body are also sensitive to the action of medicinal solutions, especially if they are rubbed in while being used internally.

a. Medicines exert a marvelously beneficial influence on nursing infants through the milk of their mother or wet nurse. Every disease of the infant yields to the homoeopathic medicine correctly chosen for the infant but given in a very moderate dose to the woman nursing him; diseases are overcome in these little ones by this method far more easily and surely than would ever be possible later on.

Since it is usually through the milk of the nurse that most infants contract psora, if they have not already inherited it from the mother, the physician can protect them from it in the same way—by medicating the milk of the nurse with an antipsoric. It is, however, absolutely necessary to treat mothers in their (first) pregnancy with a gentle antipsoric, particularly the new dynamizations of sulphur described in this edition (par. 270). This eradicates in them and in the fetus the psora, which is the cause of most chronic diseases and is almost always present in them through inheritance. In this way their offspring will be protected from it in advance. This is so true that the children of women so treated are generally born far stronger and healthier, to everybody's amazement: another confirmation of the great truth of my theory of psora.

285

The cure of very old diseases can be speeded up by daily rubbing (on back, thighs, lower legs) with the same medicinal solution found to be beneficial when taken internally. But one should of course avoid treating in this way parts affected by pains, spasms, or cutaneous eruptions.[a]

a. From this one can understand those rare miracle cures in which chronically crippled patients, whose skin was nevertheless *whole and free of disease,* speedily and permanently recover after bathing a few times in mineral baths whose medicinal constituents were by chance homoeopathic to their chronic complaint. On the other hand mineral baths *very often* make patients worse by suppressing their skin eruptions; when this happens, after a short period of well-being, the vital principle usually makes the uncured internal trouble break out in another part of the organism, one that is far more important to life and well-being, with the result, for example, that the optic nerve becomes paralyzed and amaurosis ensues or the lens becomes clouded, or hearing is lost, or insanity or asthma appear, or a stroke carries off the poor patient.

It is a cardinal principle that distinguishes the homoeopathic physician from all so-called physicians of the old school that he never uses on any of his patients a medicine whose pathological effects he has not previously determined by careful proving on the healthy (par. 20 and par. 21). To give a patient a remedy whose positive action on the health is unknown, on the basis of mere conjecture about the benefit it may perhaps have caused in some similar case or because someone says, "This remedy has helped in such and such a disease"—such an unconscionable gamble is something that the homoeopath who loves mankind leaves to the allopaths. For this reason a true physician practicing our art will *never* send his patients to any one of the innumerable mineral baths, because in almost all cases their exact positive action on human health is completely unknown, and when misused they are among the most violently dangerous remedies. Thus, among a thousand patients blindly sent to the most famous of such baths by the ignorant allopaths who have not been able to cure them, one or two come back accidentally cured, often only apparently cured, and praise the miracle to the skies, while many hundreds quietly steal home more or less aggravated, and some of them remain to prepare for the eternal resting place, a fact to which the great number of well-filled grave-yards around the most famous watering places bears witness.*

286

The dynamic forces of mineral magnetism, electricity, and galvanism act no less homoeopathically and power-fully on our vital principle than medicines actually called homoeopathic, which overcome diseases when taken by mouth, rubbed on the skin, or smelled. These other forces can cure diseases, especially those in which sensitivity and irritability are disturbed and those having abnormal sensations and involuntary muscle move-ments. But we still know far too little about the right way of using electricity, galvanism, and the so-called electromagnetic machine to put them to homoeopathic use. At least they have been used until now only pallia-tively, with great harm to patients. The positive, pure effects of electricity and galvanism on the healthy hu-man organism have not yet been thoroughly proved.

287

Magnetic power can be employed in treatment more reliably than before by the use of the positive effects of the north and south poles of a strong bar magnet, as

*Therefore a true homoeopathic physician, who never treats except on correct principles, who never risks the patient's life in a gamble where the chances of winning are one in five hundred or one in a thousand, and where losing means aggravation or death, never en-dangers any of his patients by sending them off to take their chances at a mineral bath, as allopaths often politely do to get rid of cases that they themselves or others have mismanaged.

recorded in my *Materia Medica Pura*. Both magnetic poles are equally powerful, but they are opposite to each other in their therapeutic action. The doses can be regulated by increasing or reducing the duration of application of whichever pole is indicated by the symptoms. If the effect is too violent, the application of a plate of polished zinc will serve as an antidote.

288

Here I would like to mention so-called *animal magnetism,* or *mesmerism* (as it should rather be called in gratitude to its originator, Mesmer), which differs in nature from all other medicines. This healing force, which has been frequently foolishly denied or reviled for a whole century, is a marvelous, priceless gift of God to man, by which a well-intentioned man exerts his strong will over a patient with or without touching him, or even at some distance, in such a way that the vital force of the healthy mesmerizer gifted with this power dynamically flows into the patient (as the pole of a strong bar magnet acts on a bar of unmagnetized steel). This healing force acts in different ways: on the one hand it replaces vital force in various places where it is deficient; and on the other hand it drains off, reduces, and more equally distributes it where it has become so strongly concentrated in certain parts that it has caused and sustained vague nervous conditions. It removes the general morbid derangement of the patient's vital principle and replaces it with the mesmerizer's normal one, which acts strongly on him, in such conditions as inveterate ulcers, amaurosis, paralysis of individual limbs, etc. Many sudden cures brought about at all times in history by animal magnetizers gifted with great natural power belong to this category. The most spectacular among them are those rare instances in which a man bursting with vital energy[a] uses his extremely strong and benevolent will to transmit human force to the entire organism and revive someone who has apparently been dead for some time—a sort of awakening of the dead of which history gives us many incontrovertible examples.

If the mesmerizer of either sex is capable of a benevolent enthusiasm (or even a degenerated form of it, such as bigotry, fanaticism, mysticism, or exaggerated philanthropy) he is all the more able in his charitable self-sacrifice not only to direct his forceful benevolence exclusively to the person needing it but also to concentrate it there and thus sometimes to work apparent miracles.

a. Especially one of those few who, while being very benevolent and in perfect health, *have only very slight sexual desire or none at all*. The subtle life energies that are used in all men for the production of semen are abundantly available in them and ready to be communicated by strength of will through touch to others. *All* the healing mesmerizers I have met have had this peculiar characteristic.

289

All these ways of practicing mesmerism involve the dynamic influx of a greater or lesser amount of vital energy into the patient and are termed *positive mesmerism*.[a] The way of practicing mesmerism which does the opposite is called *negative mesmerism*. The passes that are used to awaken a person from sleepwalking belong to this category, as well as all the hand movements called *calming* and *ventilating passes*. The most certain and simple of these are passes in negative mesmerism which *discharge* a surplus of vital energy that has

gathered in a single part of the organism of an undebili-
tated individual: they are effected by a very rapid
movement of the outstretched right hand held flat, ap-
proximately parallel to the surface of the body, and
about an inch above it, going from the top of the head
to the tips of the toes.[b] The more rapidly this pass is
made, the more strongly it discharges. For example, in
the apparent death of a woman, previously healthy,[c]
when her menstruation is suddenly suppressed just before its onset by a violent emotional shock, the vital
force, probably accumulated in the precordial region, is
discharged by such a rapid negative pass and redistri-
buted over the entire organism equally, so that as a
rule reanimation immediately ensues.[d] A more gentle,
less rapid negative pass can also sometimes relieve the
restlessness and anxious insomnia caused by a positive
pass that has been made too strongly on a very sensitive individual, etc.

a. When I mention here the decisive, sure healing
power of positive magnetism, I certainly do not mean
that most deplorable exaggeration of it in which repeated passes are made for a half hour or often, indeed, a whole hour at a time, day after day, to induce
in patients who have a weak nervous system that
monstrous derangement of the entire being termed
clairvoyant trance, a condition in which the person is
transported from the world of the senses and appears
to belong to the spirit world, a most dangerous and
unnatural condition by which people have often tried
in vain to cure chronic diseases.

b. It is a well-known rule that a person to be mes-
merized positively or negatively must not wear silk
anywhere on his person; but it is less well known that
the mesmerizer can communicate his vital energy

more strongly to the patient if he stands on silk than if he stands on the bare floor.

c. A negative pass, especially a very rapid one, is in any case extremely harmful to a person who is chronically weak and deficient in vitality.

d. A woman who was a self-styled magnetizer made several very strong passes one morning on a robust ten-year-old country boy for some slight indisposition, moving the tips of her thumbs along the lower edge of his ribs from the pit of the stomach to the sides. He immediately became deathly pale and fell into such a state of unconsciousness and motionlessness that he could not by any means be revived and was almost taken for dead. I had his eldest brother make a negative pass on him as rapidly as possible from the top of the head to the feet, and he immediately regained consciousness and was hale and hearty.

290

This includes to some extent the massage made by a strong and benevolent person on a patient who is slowly convalescing after being cured of a chronic disease and still suffers from emaciation, weak digestion, and lack of sleep. The individual muscles of the limbs, chest, and back are grasped and kneaded with moderate pressure. The vital principle reacts to this, restoring the tone of the muscles and their blood and lymph vessels. Of course the mesmerizing action is the main thing in this procedure, and it should not be overdone in patients who are still psychically oversensitive.

291

Baths of pure water have been found to be useful adjuvants, both palliatively and homoeopathically, in the restoration of health in acute affections and during the convalescence of patients who have just been cured of a chronic disease, when the condition of the convalescent and the temperature, duration, and frequency of the baths are properly taken into account.

But even when correctly used, baths bestow only physical benefits on the sick organism and are not in themselves really medicines. Lukewarm baths of 25 to 27 degrees Réaumur [31 to 34 degrees Centigrade] awaken the suspended irritability of tissues in apparent death from such things as freezing, drowning, or asphyxiation, where nervous sensation has been deadened. Although here such baths are only palliative, they often suffice, especially if at the same time coffee is given and the patient is rubbed by hand; and in cases where the irritability is unevenly distributed and has accumulated in certain organs, e.g., in certain hysterical and infantile convulsions, they help homoeopathically.

Similarly, in persons who have a deficiency of vital heat after being medicinally cured of a chronic disease, *momentary* immersion in cold baths of 10 to 6 degrees Réaumer [13 to 7 degrees Centigrade] has been found to be a homoeopathic adjuvant. Later, during the convalescence, *repeated,* fairly frequent immersions have been found to restore the general tonus of relaxed tissues palliatively. For this purpose they are to be given for more than a moment, often for minutes, and at increasingly cold temperatures. This is a palliative, but because it acts only physically one need not fear the counteraction that follows dynamic medicinal palliatives.

INDEX

1. Hahnemann frequently uses many different words to express exactly the same idea, for example, he speaks of removing, extinguishing, annihilating, and destroying a disease. For the sake of brevity we have sometimes indexed these different words under one word or idea that describes them all.

2. Adjectives have been indexed under the noun they qualify. A few very important ones, such as homoeopathic, allopathic, etc., have been indexed directly as well.

Index

Index

ratio, dilutant to medicine,
194, 195
Rau, 46
reaction(s)
  force, vital, of, 62, 68,
    171
  life–preserving, 62
  medicine, of, 165
  principle, vital, of, 171
  untoward, 171
record(s), 116, 179
record, to, 88, 89, 96, 115,
  119
recovery, 72, 122, 124, 127,
  169
  gradual, 101
  impediments to, 182
  incomplete, 168
  permanent, 10, 208
rectum, 13
regimen, 156, 170, 176, 180,
  182
region
  marshy (see marshy)
  precordial, 212
  swampy, 76
Reil, 36
Reine Arzneimittellehre,
  Hahnemann, 102
relatives, 59, 60, 75, 77, 84,
  90, 93, 123, 149, 155,
  159
relief, 58, 59, 76
  appearance of, 67
  immediate, 56
  palliative, 51, 52, 182
  short–lasting, 58, 61
  temporary, 53
  urgent, 136
remedy(-ies) (see also
    medicine(s)), 21, 23,

24, 91, 125, 143, 170,
  188
action(s) of, 26, 50, 98,
  140, 175
  positive, 208
  primary, 64
  secondary, 57
alternating, 40, 162
antipathic, 57, 66
antipsoric, 79, 133, 151,
  155, 156, 162
antiscabies, 40
antisyphilitic, 40, 162
appropriate, most, 10
apsoric, 156
character of, 10
choice of, 23, 152, 180
  accurate, more, 175
  appropriate, 12
  correct, 108, 175,
    183
  homoeopathic, 168
  imperfect, 136, 199
  incorrect, 176
complaints from, 199
contrary, 61, 64
dangerous, 208
disease agents as, 47
dose(s) of, 99, 130, 175,
  189
effect(s) of, 79, 202
external, 140, 141, 142,
  143, 201
favorite, 179
fevers, for, 163, 165, 166,
  167
first, 132, 151
globule of, 174
helpful, more, 179
homoeopathic, 30, 47, 52,
  64, 66, 67, 79, 96,